Quality of Anesthesia Care

Guest Editors

MARK D. NEUMAN, MD
ELIZABETH A. MARTINEZ, MD

ANESTHESIOLOGY CLINICS

www.anesthesiology.theclinics.com

Consulting Editor
LEE A. FLEISHER, MD, FACC

March 2011 • Volume 29 • Number 1

SAUNDERS an imprint of ELSEVIER, Inc.

W.B. SAUNDERS COMPANY
A Division of Elsevier Inc.

1600 John F. Kennedy Boulevard, Suite 1800 • Philadelphia, PA 19103-2899

http://www.theclinics.com

ANESTHESIOLOGY CLINICS Volume 29, Number 1
March 2011 ISSN 1932-2275, ISBN-13: 978-1-4557-0419-4

Editor: Rachel Glover
Developmental Editor: Donald E. Mumford

Anesthesiology Clinics (ISSN 1932-2275) is published quarterly by Elsevier Inc., 360 Park Avenue South, New York, NY 10010-1710. Months of issue are March, June, September, and December. Periodicals postage paid at New York, NY and at additional mailing offices. Subscription prices are $141.00 per year (US student/resident), $287.00 per year (US individuals), $351.00 per year (Canadian individuals), $459.00 per year (US institutions), $569.00 per year (Canadian institutions), $198.00 per year (Canadian and foreign student/resident), $398.00 per year (foreign individuals), and $569.00 per year (foreign institutions). To receive student and resident rate, orders must be accompanied by name of affiliated institution, date of term, and the *signature* of program/residency coordinator on institutions letterhead. Orders will be billed at individual rate until proof of status is received. Foreign air speed delivery is included in all *Clinics'* subscription prices. All prices are subject to change without notice. POSTMASTER: Send address changes to *Anesthesiology Clinics,* Elsevier Health Sciences Division, Subscription Customer Service, 3251 Riverport Lane, Maryland Heights, MO 63043. Customer Service (orders, claims, online, change of address): Elsevier Health Sciences Division, Subscription Customer Service, 3251 Riverport Lane, Maryland Heights, MO 63043. Tel:1-800-654-2452 (U.S. and Canada); 314-447-8871 (outside U.S. and Canada). Fax: 314-447-8029. E-mail: journalscustomerservice-usa@elsevier.com (for print support); journalsonlinesupport-usa@elsevier.com (for online support).

Reprints. For copies of 100 or more of articles in this publication, please contact the Commercial Reprints Department, Elsevier Inc., 360 Park Avenue South, New York, NY 10010-1710. Tel.: 212-633-3812; Fax: 212-462-1935; E-mail: reprints@elsevier.com.

Anesthesiology Clinics, is also published in Spanish by McGraw-Hill Inter-americana Editores S. A., P.O. Box 5-237, 06500 Mexico D. F., Mexico.

Anesthesiology Clinics, is covered in *MEDLINE/PubMed (Index Medicus), Current Contents/Clinical Medicine, Excerpta Medica, ISI/BIOMED,* and *Chemical Abstracts.*

Printed and bound by CPI Group (UK) Ltd, Croydon, CR0 4YY

Transferred to Digital Print 2011

Contributors

CONSULTING EDITOR

LEE A. FLEISHER, MD, FACC
Robert D. Dripps Professor and Chair of Anesthesiology and Critical Care, University of Pennsylvania School of Medicine, Philadelphia, Pennsylvania

GUEST EDITORS

MARK D. NEUMAN, MD, MSc
Assistant Professor of Anesthesiology and Critical Care, Department of Anesthesiology and Critical Care; Attending Anesthesiologist, Hospital of the University of Pennsylvania; Senior Fellow, Leonard Davis Institute for Health Economics, University of Pennsylvania, Philadelphia, Pennsylvania

ELIZABETH A. MARTINEZ, MD, MHS
Associate Professor of Anesthesia, Critical Care and Pain Medicine, Massachusetts General Hospital, Harvard University, Boston, Massachusetts

AUTHORS

MICHAEL ASHBURN, MD, MPH
Professor of Anesthesiology and Critical Care; Director, Pain Medicine and Palliative Care, Penn Pain Medicine, University of Pennsylvania, Philadelphia, Pennsylvania

REBECCA ASLAKSON, MD, MSc
Assistant Professor, Department of Anesthesiology and Critical Care Medicine, Johns Hopkins University School of Medicine, Baltimore, Maryland

JANE BALLANTYNE, MD, FRCA
Professor of Anesthesiology and Critical Care, Penn Pain Medicine Center, University of Pennsylvania, Philadelphia, Pennsylvania

SHEILA RYAN BARNETT, MD
Associate Professor of Anesthesiology, Harvard Medical School; Department of Anesthesiology, Beth Israel Deaconess Medical School, Boston, Massachusetts

ANTHONY CHAU, MD
Department of Anesthesiology, Pharmacology and Therapeutics, University of British Columbia, Vancouver, British Columbia, Canada

JESSE M. EHRENFELD, MD, MPH
Assistant Professor, Vanderbilt University; Director, Center for Evidence Based Anesthesia; Director, Perioperative Data Systems Research, Department of Anesthesiology, Vanderbilt University, Nashville, Tennessee

ADAM S. EVANS, MD, MBA
Critical Care Fellow, Department of Anesthesiology, New York-Presbyterian Hospital, Columbia Presbyterian Medical Center, New York, New York

SUSAN L. FAGGIANI, RN, BA, CPHQ
Regulatory Administrator, Department of Anesthesiology, New York-Presbyterian Hospital, Weill Cornell Medical College; Quality and Patient Safety Liaison, Housestaff Quality Council, New York-Presbyterian Hospital, New York, New York

PETER M. FLEISCHUT, MD
Assistant Professor of Anesthesiology, Department of Anesthesiology, Weill Cornell Medical College; Deputy Quality and Patient Safety Officer, New York-Presbyterian Hospital, New York, New York

ALLAN FRANKEL, MD
Principal, Pascal Metrics Inc, Washington, DC

ANITA GUPTA, DO, PharmD
Assistant Professor of Anesthesiology and Critical Care, Penn Pain Medicine Center, University of Pennsylvania, Philadelphia, Pennsylvania

GEORGE M. HANNA, MD
Resident Physician, Department of Anesthesia, Critical Care and Pain Medicine, Massachusetts General Hospital; Clinical Fellow in Anesthesia, Harvard Medical School, Boston, Massachusetts

ROBERT E. HODY, BSEE, MSEE, MSCS
Lean Kaizen Internal Consultant, Johns Hopkins Medicine, Center for Innovation in Quality Patient Care, Baltimore, Maryland

STEPHANIE B. JONES, MD
Associate Professor of Anaesthesia, Harvard Medical School; Residency Program Director and Vice Chair for Education, Department of Anesthesia, Critical Care and Pain Medicine, Beth Israel Deaconess Medical Center, Boston, Massachusetts

GREGORY E. KERR, MD, MBA
Associate Professor of Clinical Anesthesiology, Department of Anesthesiology, Weill Cornell Medical College; Medical Director, Critical Care Services; Faculty Advisor, Housestaff Quality Council, New York-Presbyterian Hospital, New York, New York

SACHIN KHETERPAL, MD, MBA
Department of Anesthesiology, University of Michigan Medical School, Ann Arbor, Michigan

RIKANTE KVERAGA, MD
Instructor in Anesthesia, Harvard Medical School; Staff Anesthesiologist, Department of Anesthesia, Critical Care and Pain Medicine, Beth Israel Deaconess Medical Center, Boston, Massachusetts

ELIOT J. LAZAR, MD, MBA
Associate Professor of Clinical Medicine, Department of Medicine; Associate Professor of Clinical Public Health, Department of Public Health, Weill Cornell Medical College; Senior Vice President and Chief Quality and Patient Safety Officer, New York-Presbyterian Hospital, New York, New York

WILTON C. LEVINE, MD
Attending Anesthesiologist and Clinical Director, Department of Anesthesia, Critical Care and Pain Medicine, Massachusetts General Hospital; Assistant Professor of Anesthesia, Harvard Medical School, Boston, Massachusetts

ELIZABETH A. MARTINEZ, MD, MHS
Associate Professor of Anesthesia, Critical Care and Pain Medicine, Massachusetts General Hospital, Harvard University, Boston, Massachusetts

JOHN MCGREADY, PhD, MS
Assistant Scientist, Department of Biostatistics, Johns Hopkins Bloomberg School of Public Health, Baltimore, Maryland

ALEJANDRO J. NECOCHEA, MD, MPH
Instructor, Department of Internal Medicine, Johns Hopkins University School of Medicine, Baltimore, Maryland

MICHAEL NUROK, MD, PhD
Department of Anesthesiology, Perioperative and Pain Medicine, Brigham and Women's Hospital, Boston, Massachusetts; Hospital for Special Surgery, New York, New York

CHRISTINE S. PARK, MD
Assistant Professor, Department of Anesthesiology; Assistant Professor, Institute for Healthcare Studies; Medical Director, Northwestern Center for Clinical Simulation, Northwestern University Feinberg School of Medicine, Chicago, Illinois

JULIUS C. PHAM, MD, PhD
Department of Emergency Medicine, Department of Anesthesia and Critical Care Medicine, Quality and Safety Research Group, Johns Hopkins University School of Medicine, Baltimore, Maryland

PETER J. PRONOVOST, MD, PhD
Professor, Department of Anesthesiology and Critical Care Medicine, Johns Hopkins University School of Medicine, Baltimore, Maryland

SATYA KRISHNA RAMACHANDRAN, MD, FRCA
Department of Anesthesiology, University of Michigan Medical School, Ann Arbor, Michigan

BRIAN ROTHMAN, MD
Assistant Professor of Anesthesiology; Director, Perioperative Informatics, Vanderbilt University School of Medicine, Nashville, Tennessee

WARREN S. SANDBERG, MD, PhD
Professor of Anesthesiology, Surgery and Biomedical Informatics; Chair, Department of Anesthesiology, Vanderbilt University School of Medicine, Nashville, Tennessee

FREDERICK E. SIEBER, MD
Director of Anesthesiology and Clinical Research, Department of Anesthesiology, Johns Hopkins Bayview Medical Center; Associate Professor, Anesthesiology and Critical Care Medicine, Johns Hopkins University School of Medicine, Baltimore, Maryland

PAUL ST JACQUES, MD
Associate Professor of Anesthesiology, Anesthesia Patient Safety Officer, Department of Anesthesiology, Vanderbilt University School of Medicine, Nashville, Tennessee

JERRY STONEMETZ, MD
Clinical Associate, Anesthesia and Critical Care Medicine, Johns Hopkins University School of Medicine, Baltimore, Maryland

THORALF M. SUNDT III, MD
Division of Cardiovascular Surgery, Mayo Clinic, Rochester, Minnesota

Contents

The literature defining and addressing teamwork and communication is abundant; however, few studies have analyzed the relationship between measures of teamwork and communication and quantifiable outcomes. The objectives of this review are: (1) to identify studies addressing teamwork and communication in the operating room in relation to discrete measures of outcome, (2) to create a classification of studies of the relationship between teamwork and communication and outcomes, (3) to assess the implications of these studies, (4) to explore the methodological challenges of teamwork and communication studies in the perioperative setting, and (5) to suggest future research directions.

Simulation, a strategy for improving the quality and safety of patient care, is used for the training of technical and nontechnical skills and for training in teamwork and communication. This article reviews simulation-based research, with a focus on anesthesiology, at 3 different levels of outcome: (1) as measured in the simulation laboratory, (2) as measured in clinical performance, and (3) as measured in patient outcomes. It concludes with a discussion of some current uses of simulation, which include the identification of latent failures and the role of simulation in continuing professional practice assessment for anesthesiologists.

This article summarizes the current state of technology as it pertains to quality in the operating room, ties the current state back to its evolutionary pathway to understand how the current capabilities and their limitations came to pass, and elucidates how the overlay of information technology (IT) as a wrapper around current monitoring and device technology provides a significant advance in the ability of anesthesiologists to use technology to improve quality along many axes. The authors posit that IT will enable all the information about patients, perioperative systems, system capacity, and readiness to follow a development trajectory of increasing usefulness.

Anesthesia information management systems (AIMS) are becoming more commonplace in operating rooms across the world and have the potential to help clinicians measure and improve perioperative quality. However, to realize the full potential of AIMS, clinicians must first understand their capabilities and limitations. This article reviews the literature on AIMS, focusing on areas where AIMS have been shown to have a meaningful impact on quality, safety, and operational efficiency.

The challenges to prospective randomized controlled trials have necessitated the exploration of observational data sets that support research into the predictors and modulators of preoperative adverse events. The primary purpose and design of quality improvement databases is quality assessment and improvement at the local, regional, or national level. However, these data can also provide the opportunity to robustly study specific questions related to patient outcomes with no additional clinical risk to the patient. The virtual explosion of anesthesia-related registries has opened seemingly limitless opportunities for outcomes research in addition to generating hypothesis for more rigorous prospective analysis.

Postoperative complications are directly related to poor surgical outcomes in the elderly. This review outlines evidence based quality initiatives focused on decreasing neurologic, cardiac, and pulmonary complications in the elderly surgical patient. Important anesthesia quality initiatives for prevention of delirium, the most common neurologic complication in elderly surgical patients, are outlined. There are few age-specific quality measures aimed at prevention of cardiac and pulmonary complications. However, some recommendations for adults can be applied to the geriatric surgical population. In the future, process measures may provide a more global assessment of quality in the elderly surgical population.

Multidisciplinary education (MDE) is perceived as the next means of implementing major improvements in the quality and cost-effectiveness of patient care. In this article, the authors discuss various definitions of MDE, evaluate how MDE might be implemented in clinical arenas relevant to the anesthesiologist, and describe several implementations of MDE within their hospital and the anesthesiology department.

and procedure creation, and culture change was led by the Department of Anesthesiology of the Weill Medical College of Cornell University. A Housestaff Quality Council was started in 2008 that has partnered with hospital leadership and clinical departments to engage the housestaff in quality and patient safety initiatives, resulting in measurable improvements in several patient care projects and enhanced working relationships among various clinical constituencies. Ultimately this attempt to change culture has found great success in fostering a relationship between the housestaff and the hospital in ways that have and will continue to improve patient care.

VISIT US ONLINE!
Access your subscription at:
www.theclinics.com

Foreword

Quality of Anesthesia Care

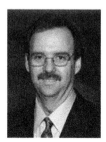

Lee A. Fleisher, MD
Consulting Editor

For the past decade, there has been an interest in focusing on the quality of care delivered as opposed to just the quantity of care. Part of this focus relates to several Institute of Medicine reports, the first of which focused on safety and the second on quality. The rationale for improving quality of care is obvious from a patient perspective, but there is also an economic imperative since higher quality may actually decrease costs. As part of the health care reform debate and legislation in the United States, there has been a focus on value-based purchasing including the development of incentives for achieving "quality." However, there continues to be debate as to the measurement of quality in different venues and the means to achieve these goals. It is within this context that an issue of *Anesthesiology Clinics* was developed.

In deciding to devote an issue to quality and identifying leaders in this area, I have been fortunate to attract two rising stars in the area of researching quality. Both Mark D. Neuman, MD, MS, and Elizabeth A. Martinez, MD, MHS have developed academic careers in this area. They are also both members of the Committee on Performance and Outcomes Measurement of the American Society of Anesthesiologists, the group tasked to develop performance measurement. Mark D. Neuman is currently an Assistant Professor of Anesthesiology and Critical Care at the University of Pennsylvania School of Medicine. After a residency in anesthesiology at the Brigham and Women's Hospital, he completed a Robert Wood Johnson Clinical Scholar Program and Master of Science in Health Policy Research at Penn. He has already published several important articles on the care of patients undergoing repair of a hip fracture. Elizabeth A. Martinez is currently an Associate Professor of Anesthesia, Critical Care and Pain Medicine at the Massachusetts General Hospital. She completed her residency in anesthesiology and fellowships in critical care and cardiac anesthesia at The Johns Hopkins Hospital and remained on the faculty for several years. She is completing a grant on Organization of Care and Outcomes in Cardiac Surgery from the Agency for Healthcare Research and Quality and is starting another on Developing and Testing

Anesthesiology Clin 29 (2011) xiii–xiv
doi:10.1016/j.anclin.2010.12.002   **anesthesiology.theclinics.com**

a Set of Measures to Assess Safety in High-Risk Intensive Care Units from The Commonwealth Fund. Together, they solicited outstanding individuals to educate us on this important topic.

Lee A. Fleisher, MD
University of Pennsylvania School of Medicine
3400 Spruce Street, Dulles 680
Philadelphia, PA 19104, USA

E-mail address:
lee.fleisher@uphs.upenn.edu

Preface

Finding the Fourth Branch— Understanding Quality-of-Care in Anesthesiology

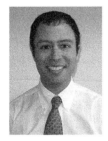 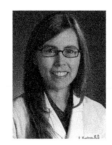

Mark D. Neuman, MD, MSc   Elizabeth A. Martinez, MD, MHS
Guest Editors

Writing in 1934, Robert Hutchison described "the three great branches of clinical science—diagnosis, prognosis, and treatment."[1] Today, while none of these three tasks have diminished in importance, physicians, along with the consumers, purchasers, and regulators of health care in the United States, have come to recognize the responsibility to measure and improve quality in health care as a fourth, essential branch of contemporary medical practice.

The growing recognition of gaps in the quality and safety of health care provided in the U.S.—crystallized by two landmark reports by the Institute of Medicine, *To Err is Human*[2] and *Crossing the Quality Chasm*[3]—has sparked a growing recognition that health care in the U.S. falls short of meeting standards most would accept as "high quality." These works, as well as findings that patients with chronic diseases in the U.S. receive evidence-based care only 55% of the time,[4] has fueled conversations over the past decade regarding the way health care is organized, regulated, and reimbursed.

Medicare, the largest single payer within the U.S. health care economy, now monitors hospital performance on selected outcomes of care, making comparisons between hospitals public via the Web. Further, to provide incentives for physicians and other health care professionals to improve the care they deliver, Medicare has defined a set of "never events"—potentially preventable occurrences whose costs will no longer be reimbursed by Medicare.[5] In addition, the Medicare Modernization Act of 2004 has mandated that Medicare institute a system of "pay-for-performance," seeking to link payments to hospitals and physicians directly to the quality of services they provide to the health care consumer.[6]

For anesthesiologists, understanding their place within the landscape of health care quality improvement is a complex challenge. The multifaceted nature of our specialty,

Anesthesiology Clin 29 (2011) xv–xx
doi:10.1016/j.anclin.2010.12.001   **anesthesiology.theclinics.com**
1932-2275/11/$ – see front matter

with care occurring in operating rooms, intensive care suites, labor floors, and pain clinics, and the diversity of the patients we serve, ranging from neonates to the oldest-of-old, confound simple definitions of high-quality anesthesia care. Further, the frequent presence of anesthesiologists within larger teams of physicians, nurses, and other professionals often makes it difficult to identify the contribution of the anesthesiologist to patient outcomes. Such challenges are compounded by important gaps in evidence surrounding fundamental aspects of anesthesia practice, along with our still limited understanding of how to systematically record and evaluate the quality of the care delivered by anesthesiologists.

The present issue of *Anesthesiology Clinics* represents an introduction to current efforts of leaders in anesthesiology to confront some of these challenges. In particular, we have sought in assembling this volume to portray a variety of perspectives on quality improvement within anesthesiology across a range of practice settings and patient populations. More fundamentally, though, the articles in this volume speak to the multiple definitions of "quality" that exist for physicians practicing in our specialty, which range from efforts to improve care at the bedside for patients at the end of life within the ICU, to efforts to improve processes on a large scale at the level of health care systems.

While a number of these articles touch on topics specific to the everyday practice of anesthesia, such as care of the older operative patient or communication within the operating room, each of these articles has been included as a means of illustrating parts of a larger framework shared by research on quality measurement and improvement across medical care. As a means of introduction to the articles presented here, as well as the science of quality more generally, we briefly review here a number of these key principles of quality in health care.

WHAT IS QUALITY IN HEALTH CARE?

Before we can discuss efforts that are focused on measuring and improving the quality of health care, we must identify a uniform definition of what constitutes quality. As a fundamental step toward defining basic characteristics of quality in health care, the Institute of Medicine's 2001 report, *Crossing the Quality Chasm,*[3] proposes six aims to define what "health care should be" (**Box 1**).

For the present discussion, and for most efforts at quality improvement, these six aims—*safety, effectiveness, patient-centeredness, timeliness, efficiency,* and *equity*—constitute a working definition of quality in health care that we will use.

The measurement of performance in health care represents a longstanding, fundamental aspect of any effort to improve care. In 1911, Massachusetts General Hospital surgeon Ernest Codman established an "end results system" to monitor his own patients' outcomes with the goal of improving the care he and his colleagues delivered in the future.[7,8] These efforts ultimately led to the development of the Hospital Standardization Program, known today as The Joint Commission, the foremost accrediting body of health care organizations worldwide.

Alongside the external review mechanism provided by The Joint Commission, the majority of initial and ongoing efforts by individual anesthesiologists and anesthesiology departments to improve quality are through reviews of adverse events through peer review, morbidity and mortality conferences, isolated liability claims, and incident reports.[9] However, these mechanisms frequently did not allow for systematic learning, such as what was first introduced by Codman.

More recently, such individual and departmental efforts to monitor the quality of health care have given rise to larger scale initiatives to systematically learn from

---

Box 1
Six attributes of a High-Quality Health Care System[3]

1. Safety

   Avoids injuries to patients from the care that is intended to help them.

2. Effectiveness

   Provides services based on scientific knowledge to all who could benefit and refrains from providing services to those not likely to benefit.

3. Patient-centeredness

   Provides care that is respectful and responsive to individual patient preferences, needs, and values and ensures that patient values guide all clinical decisions.

4. Timeliness

   Reduces waits and sometimes harmful delays for both those who receive and those who give care.

5. Efficiency

   Avoids waste, including waste of equipment, supplies, ideas, and energy.

6. Equity

   Provides care that does not vary in quality because of personal characteristics such as gender, ethnicity, geographic location, or socioeconomic status.

---

gaps in quality and translate these lessons to improvements in patient outcomes. As a result, current efforts to measure and broadly improve the quality of care have required the development of a generalizable framework to organize the evaluation and improvement of care.

A FRAMEWORK FOR MONITORING QUALITY

Writing in 1988, Avedis Donabedian introduced a summary of his efforts to answering the question of how to assess the quality of health care:

> There was a time, not too long ago, when this question could not have been asked. The quality of care was considered to be something of a mystery: real capable of being perceived and appreciated, but not subject to measurement. The very attempt to define and measure quality seemed, then, to denature and belittle it. Now, we may have moved too far in the opposite direction. Those who have not experienced the intricacies of clinical practice demand measures that are easy, precise, and complete—as if a sack of potatoes was being weighed. True, some elements in the quality of care are easy to define and measure, but there are also profundities that still elude us. We must not allow anyone to belittle or ignore them; they are the secret and glory of our art. Therefore, we should avoid claiming for our capacity to assess quality either too little or too much.[10]

Donabedian's comments more than two decades ago remain relevant for a range of efforts to define and measure quality in health care and carry a special resonance for fields that, like anesthesiology, are at an early stage of the systematic examination and improvement of care. Indeed, the articles we have collected in this volume each can be viewed within Donabedian's own concepts of structure, process, and outcome, which we outline in **Table 1**.

Table 1	
Donabedian's Framework for measuring Quality in Health Care[10]	
Domain	**Example/Description**
Structure	The attributes of the settings in which care occurs, including material resources, human resources, organizational structure, and technology
Process	What is actually done in giving and receiving care, both by the patient and by the health care provider in terms of evaluation, diagnosis, and therapy
Outcome	The effects of care on patient well-being and satisfaction with care

At the same time they all share an acknowledgment of "the profundities that still elude us" in evaluating the practice of clinical anesthesia, and as such, can be read as efforts to demarcate what is known about quality from what has yet to be elucidated.[10]

The framework proposed by Donabedian remains the dominant paradigm through which we understand quality measurement and quality improvement in health care; at its core, it describes three domains within which the quality of health care can be evaluated. These domains are structure, process, and outcomes and are described in **Table 1**.

Importantly, these three categories are interdependent, with good outcomes predicated on high-quality processes of care, which are, in turn, reliant on high-quality structures for care delivery. As a consequence, the logic of quality measurement in these domains is wedded to such an interlinked structure: assessments of the structure of health care require evidence of a clear link to better performance in processes of care known to produce good outcomes; assessments of the processes of health care are dependent on knowledge of a meaningful effect of processes on outcomes. Furthermore, assessments of outcomes, such as mortality, complications, or rehospitalizations, are only truly meaningful for quality improvement when they serve to identify a gap in the quality of health care structures or processes amenable to intervention.

IMPLEMENTING QUALITY IMPROVEMENT

While the authors in this volume of *Anesthesiology Clinics* report on their successful implementation of quality improvement programs, we need to acknowledge that this is no easy feat. In the next section we very briefly highlight some key considerations for the successful implementation of both large and small quality improvement (QI) initiatives.

Collaborating to Improve

As we have found in our own efforts to improve the safety of care delivered in our own institutions, punitive approaches to errors in care frequently fail to actually prevent future errors or improve patient outcomes. Importantly, approaches that punish individual physicians for shortcomings in care may only serve to reinforce barriers to disclosure of errors and evaluation of flawed processes, preventing future improvement. Instead, we have emphasized the need to engage physicians in efforts to find ways to improve care delivery through education, technology, and teamwork. The articles in this volume each reflect this aspect of quality improvement, which we envision as an important component in driving progress toward better delivery of health care.

Measuring Our Processes and Outcomes

An ability to measure performance is a prerequisite to improving performance. Historically, for anesthesiologists, a lack of access to retrospective data on processes and outcomes of care represented an important barrier to improving care. In the present volume, two articles point to the potential for automated anesthesia information systems (AIMS) to allow a wide group of practices to improve their collective learning from data feedback. Indeed, AIMs solve a crucial problem for QI initiatives in anesthesiology—integrating data collection relevant to quality improvement into the already complex workflow of daily practice is an imperative first step. The American Society of Anesthesiologists has recognized the potential for AIMs to serve as a quality-improvement tool and has created the Anesthesia Quality Institute (AQI). A stated goal of the AQI is to gather patient data from anesthesia programs nationally for the development of a national anesthesia outcomes registry. This will serve to allow for benchmarking anesthesia providers across structure and process measures in addition to outcomes and importantly to potentially identify best practices and drive future comparative effectiveness research in anesthesia.

Finding Leaders

Leaders for quality improvement efforts may emerge from, and should be sought within, all levels of a health care organization. As Fleischut and colleagues point out in this volume's article on resident trainee leadership in quality improvement, front-line staff may serve key roles as "champions" for quality improvement. Indeed, we have found efforts involving alliances between high-level institutional leadership and front-line staff to be more successful than initiatives led by either of such groups in isolation.

Identifying and Overcoming Barriers

We acknowledge that changing physician behavior is very difficult, and a broad literature exists on barriers to changing the way doctors practice medicine.[11] Further, the most important barriers to change may frequently be local phenomena, such as aspects of hospital culture that can only be identified and addressed at a local level. Identifying such barriers serves as a fundamental first step toward development of strategies to overcome them in efforts to improve quality. Gurses and colleagues have developed an instrument to identify local barriers.[12]

SUMMARY

The "fourth branch" of clinical practice in anesthesiology—to measure and improve the quality of care we deliver—remains a young and continuously evolving science. In assembling this volume of *Anesthesiology Clinics*, we have sought to capture some of the diverse challenges and innovations leaders in our field have made to evaluate and improve the care we currently provide. We view all of these contributions as an expression of the collective "continuous learning" of our specialty, and a recognition that true quality improvement requires discourse about both failures and successes in care improvement efforts. We thus offer these articles as both academic reports and notes from the front that may offer some insight in helping disseminate new ideas for how to improve anesthesia quality at both the local and the national level.

Mark D. Neuman, MD, MSc
Department of Anesthesiology and Critical Care
University of Pennsylvania
1117 Blockley Hall
423 Guardian Drive
Philadelphia, PA 19104, USA

Elizabeth A. Martinez, MD, MHS
Department of Anesthesia, Critical Care and Pain Medicine
Massachusetts General Hospital
Harvard University
55 Fruit Street
Boston, MA 02114, USA

E-mail addresses:
neumanm@mail.med.upenn.edu (M.D. Neuman)
emartinez10@partners.org (E.A. Martinez)

REFERENCES

1. Hutchinson RM. Prognosis. Lancet 1934;1:697–8.
2. Kohn LT, Corrigan JM, Donaldson MS, editors. To err is human: building a safer health system. Washington, DC: National Academy Press; 2000.
3. Institute of Medicine (U.S.). Committee on Quality of Health Care in America. Crossing the quality chasm: a new health system for the 21st century. Washington, DC: National Academy Press; 2001.
4. McGlynn EA, Asch SM, Adams J, et al. The quality of health care delivered to adults in the United States. N Engl J Med 2003;348(26):2635–45.
5. Milstein A. Ending extra payment for "never events"—stronger incentives for patients' safety. N Engl J Med 2009;360(23):2388–90.
6. Epstein AM. Paying for performance in the United States and abroad. N Engl J Med 2006;355(4):406–8.
7. Donabedian A. The end results of health care: Ernest Codman's contribution to quality assessment and beyond. Milbank Q 1989;67(2):233–56 [discussion: 257–67].
8. Noble J. The Codman competition: rewarding excellence in performance measurement, 19–20. Jt Comm J Qual Patient Saf 2006;32(11):634–40.
9. Miller RD. Miller's anesthesia. 7th edition. Philadelphia (PA): Churchill Livingstone/ Elsevier; 2009.
10. Donabedian A. The quality of care—how can it be assessed. JAMA 1988; 260(12):1743–8.
11. Cabana MD, Rand CS, Powe NR, et al. Why don't physicians follow clinical practice guidelines? A framework for improvement. JAMA 1999;282(15):1458–65.
12. Gurses AP, Murphy DJ, Martinez EA, et al. A practical tool to identify and eliminate barriers to compliance with evidence-based guidelines. Jt Comm J Qual Patient Saf 2009;35(10):526–32, 485.

Teamwork and Communication in the Operating Room: Relationship to Discrete Outcomes and Research Challenges

Michael Nurok, MD, PhD[a,b,]*, Thoralf M. Sundt III, MD[c],
Allan Frankel, MD[d]

KEYWORDS

- Teamwork • Communication • Outcomes • Perioperative
- Surgery • Operating room • Behavior

There has been considerable interest in defining and measuring teamwork and communication in the perioperative setting. The goal of this work has been to develop metrics of teamwork and communication with a view to measuring the effect of interventions to improve perioperative teamwork and communication. Although the literature on teamwork and communication is abundant, few studies have analyzed the relationship between measures of teamwork and communication and other quantifiable outcomes. This limitation is particularly pertinent to simulation-based studies, which by definition cannot measure quantifiable outcomes in real practice. The objectives of the current review are (1) to identify studies addressing teamwork and communication in the operating room in relation to discrete measures of outcome, (2) to create a classification of studies on the relationship between teamwork and communication and outcomes, (3) to assess the implications of these studies, (4) to explore

Disclosures: Allan Frankel is a Principal at Pascal Metrics, a software analytics and consulting group aimed at data-driven interventions to improve patient safety and risk management.
[a] Department of Anesthesiology, Hospital for Special Surgery, 535 East 70th Street, New York, NY 10021, USA
[b] Department of Anesthesiology, Brigham and Women's Hospital, Boston, MA, USA
[c] Division of Cardiovascular Surgery, Mayo Clinic, 200 First Street SW, Rochester, MN 55905, USA
[d] Pascal Metrics Inc, 3050 K Street NW, Suite 205, Washington, DC, USA
* Corresponding author.
E-mail address: nurokm@hss.edu

Anesthesiology Clin 29 (2011) 1–11
doi:10.1016/j.anclin.2010.11.012   **anesthesiology.theclinics.com**
1932-2275/11/$ – see front matter © 2011 Elsevier Inc. All rights reserved.

the methodological challenges of teamwork and communication studies in the perioperative setting, and (5) to suggest future research directions.

METHODS

A literature search was performed using the National Library of Medicine catalog and the following 3 search strategies, (((((Teamwork) OR Communication) OR Behavior) AND Surgery) AND Operating Room) AND (Outcome OR Error), (((Teamwork) AND Communication) AND Operating Room), and (((Teamwork) AND Communication) AND Surgery).

In total, 246 articles were returned. Criteria for inclusion in this study were that the article (1) addressed teamwork and/or communication in the operating room and (2) reported an outcome. Criteria for exclusion were that the article was (1) a review (2) a pure methods article (3) a pure survey of attitudes or perception (4) based on simulation, (5) based on a checklist approach. Based on these criteria, 8 studies were identified.

RESULTS
Clinical Outcomes

Outcome measures used to assess the effect of measured teamwork and communication in the operating room include morbidity, mortality, technical errors, operating time and delays, and communication failures (**Table 1**). These outcomes have been measured directly or by proxy. In addition, some studies report risk factors for poor outcomes related to teamwork and communication. Various definitions and measurements of teamwork and communication themselves have been used in these studies.

Table 1
Outcome measures used in identified studies

References	Morbidity and/ or Mortality	Technical Errors	Operating Times and Delays	Teamwork and/or Communication Failures
Catchpole et al,[4] 2008	—	X	X	—
Davenport et al,[1] 2007	X	—	—	—
El Bardissi et al,[5] 2008	—	X	—	X
Lingard et al,[8] 2004	—	—	—	X
Mazzocco et al,[2] 2009	X	—	—	—
Nielsen et al,[3] 2007	X	—	—	—
Nurok et al,[9] 2010	—	—	—	X
Wiegmann et al,[6] 2007	—	X	—	X

X is a measurement in this study.

Risk-adjusted morbidity and mortality
The authors identified 3 studies that evaluated a relationship between measures of teamwork and communication and risk-adjusted morbidity or mortality. Davenport and colleagues[1] used an organizational climate safety survey (a questionnaire that measures the respondent's perception of an organization's safety climate) of 52 sites, receiving 6083 responses (response rate 52%), but they could not correlate the survey results with the National Surgical Quality Improvement Program (a nationally validated risk-adjusted morbidity and mortality data program to measure and improve the quality of surgical care). However, they did find that the reported levels of communication with attending and resident physicians correlated with the risk-adjusted morbidity.

Mazzocco and colleagues[2] used a standardized observation instrument to measure perioperative team behaviors during 293 operative procedures. The instrument used operational definitions of briefing, information sharing, inquiry, assertion, vigilance and awareness, and contingency management. The observers rated how often behaviors were observed. A retrospective chart review was then performed to measure the 30-day outcome. Results were adjusted by the American Society of Anesthesiologists score. Patients undergoing operations by teams demonstrating less-frequent measured information sharing during intraoperative phases, briefing during hand off phases, and information sharing during hand off phases had increased odds of complication or death. Composite measures of inadequate teamwork behaviors were also positively associated with increased odds of death or complication.

Nielsen and colleagues[3] conducted a randomized controlled trial at 15 obstetric centers (7 intervention, 8 control) involving implementation of a curriculum focusing on measures of communication and team structure. The primary outcome was a composite score of adverse maternal and neonatal outcomes, including death. The study did not find a relationship between the composite score of adverse outcome and the intervention.

Technical errors
Several studies used technical errors as a measurable outcome. Catchpole and colleagues[4] observed 26 laparoscopic cholecystectomies and 22 carotid endarterectomies, scoring team skills for the entire team and the nursing, surgical, and anesthetic subteams using a standardized observation instrument. The instrument measured team skills for leadership and management, teamwork and cooperation, problem solving and decision making, and situation awareness. These skills were rated on a range from below standard to excellent. The investigators found that errors in surgical technique had a strong association with surgical situation awareness.

El Bardissi and colleagues[5] conducted an observational study of 31 cardiac surgical cases. Recorded data included teamwork failures, technical errors, and team structure. A correlation was found between teamwork failures and technical errors (defined as technical events in which a planned sequence of activities failed to initially achieve its intended outcome). Teams consisting of members familiar with the operating surgeon had significantly fewer event failures compared with teams that did not have such members.

The same group of investigators analyzed flow disruptions (any issue in teamwork, technology/instruments, training, or the environment that results in deviation from the natural progression of an operation, thereby potentially compromising safety) in cardiac surgical cases over a 3-week period. Surgical errors increased with flow disruptions, and teamwork and communication failures were the strongest predictors of these errors.[6] None of these errors, however, resulted in adverse events.

Operating times and delays

The relationship between teamwork and communication and operating times and/or delays has also been investigated. Catchpole and colleagues[4] in their above-cited study of laparoscopic cholecystectomies and carotid endarterectomies found that the operating time decreased with higher leadership and management scores for surgical teams but increased with higher leadership and management skills for anesthesia teams. This latter result was because of the longer duration of carotid endarterectomies. The investigators attributed the increased procedural length to the complexity of the cases and speculated that greater anesthetic leadership and management skills were required to safely manage these patients.

Communication failures

Several studies have examined communication failure as an outcome. Amongst the outcomes measured by El Bardissi and colleagues[5] were procedural information failures and failures caused by hand offs. Of note, there were fewer total event failures when team members were familiar with the operating surgeon.

In a study by Lingard and colleagues,[7] trained observers recorded 90 hours of observations over 48 surgical procedures. Of 421 communication events recorded, 129 were categorized as failures, including poor timing, missing or inaccurate information, unresolved issues, and exclusion of key individuals. One-third of these failures were thought to result in effects that jeopardized patient safety by increasing cognitive load, interrupting routine, and increasing tension in the operating room.

Nurok and colleagues[8] used a standardized observation instrument to record various phases of complex thoracic surgical procedures before and after two 90-minute teamwork-training interventions with the involved surgeons, anesthesiologists, and nursing staff. Measured teamwork outcomes before and after the training intervention included a calculated score of teamwork and communication, which included failures in communication. The second main outcome was termed "threat-to-patient outcome" a composite index of factors commonly thought to increase the risk of adverse perioperative outcomes. After the teamwork-training intervention, the calculated teamwork and communication scores improved and the calculated threat to patient outcome score decreased; this result was durable for the threat-to-patient outcome.

Study Methods

Various methods have been used to measure outcomes in relation to teamwork and communication (**Table 2**). By far, the most common method is direct observation; however, others include the use of standardized instruments, quantitative and qualitative analyses of recorded observation, anonymous reporting, review of adverse events and root cause analysis, and surveys in conjunction with these measurements. An example of an observation instrument can be found in **Figs. 1** and **2**.

Some of the studies cited in this review included behavioral interventions. These interventions included nonspecific educational sessions with subjects and teamwork-training sessions and audits with feedback. Studies using checklists to ensure implementation of clinical pathways, protocols, or guidelines were excluded.

DISCUSSION
Implications of Research on Teamwork and Communication in Relationship to Perioperative Outcomes

There is growing consensus that teamwork and communication failures contribute to perioperative adverse events; however, there are few data supporting this assertion.

| | | | Survey | |
References	Direct Observation	Standardized Instrument	with Other Data	Intervention
Catchpole et al,[4] 2008	X	X	—	—
Davenport et al,[1] 2007	—	—	X	—
El Bardissi et al,[5] 2008	X	—	—	—
Lingard et al,[8] 2004	X	—	—	—
Mazzocco et al,[2] 2009	X	X	—	—
Nielsen et al,[3] 2007	—	—	—	X
Nurok et al,[9] 2009	X	X	—	X
Wiegmann et al,[6] 2007	X	—	—	—

Table 2
Methods used in identified studies

X is a measurement in this study.

The authors could find only 3 studies attempting to identify a relationship between measures of teamwork and communication and perioperative morbidity and mortality.[1–3] Only one of these studies identified a significantly increased risk of death in the setting of infrequent information sharing.[2] The remaining studies that were identified reported relationships between measures of teamwork and communication and outcomes that were harder to consistently quantify or less frequently reported, including technical errors, operating times and delays, communication failures, and other adverse events.

There are more data supporting a relationship between teamwork and communication and other outcomes such as technical failures.[4] It is logical that technical failures represent a potential risk for morbidity and/or mortality; however, objective demonstration of the same is lacking. One study has identified a relationship between operative times or delays and teamwork and communication.[4] More data are needed to explore these relationships.

Most studies of teamwork and communication have used indices of teamwork and communication themselves as outcomes. The challenge of these studies is to relate measurements of teamwork and communication to harder outcomes that are more relevant to patient care.

As a whole, this body of literature weakly demonstrates relationships between teamwork and communication and measured outcomes. It is unclear whether the weakness of these relationships is because of the methodological challenges of the research or the true absence of a strong relationship. Continued research in this domain is worthwhile because even small new insights will influence what health care systems currently do to optimize perioperative clinicians' teamwork and communication skills and also because of the pervasive view that communication and teamwork failures play a large role in most severe perioperative adverse events, suggesting an effect that has not been adequately measured. For these reasons, understanding the methodological challenges and optimizing the approaches to teamwork and communication research will be critical to future studies.

Methodological challenges of teamwork and communication research in the operating room

There are multiple methodological challenges in performing perioperative teamwork and communication research aimed at measuring discrete outcomes, including the

Communication, Teamwork, Threats and Climate Assessment

Observer ID: _____ Observation Start Time:_____ Expected Sheet Change at: _____ (10 minutes from Start Time) Sheet #:_____

Complete for first sheet only

1

Project Time period: Pre-training / Post-training / Sustaining **Day of the Week:** Monday-Friday / Weekend / Holiday

Procedure:_____ ASA Classification: _____ Patient age: <40 40-60 >60 Patient Gender: (M) (F)

Attending surgeon in room: Y / N   Attending Anesthesiologist in room: Y / N

Circle reason(s) for sheet change

2

1: First sheet of observation

2: 10 minutes expired

3: Climate Changed in one of the Three Areas, please indicate cause below:

(Inconsistent Behavior) (Change in Vital Signs) (Bleeding) (Equipment Problem) (Critical Portion of Procedure) (Other_____)

3

Segment of Procedure (check one)

Patient entering room___ Induction___ Prep and Drape____ Incision_____ Intra Op ___ Closing ___ Patient waking up ___

If critical portion of procedure please describe _____

Vital Signs: BP_____ MAP _____ HR_____ O₂Sat_____

Climate Score: Assess when starting this sheet

Area 1 = surgical and sterile environment	(1)Disengaged	(2)Engaged	(3)Appropriately Tense	(4)Inappropriately Tense
Area 2 = anesthetic environment	(1)Disengaged	(2)Engaged	(3)Appropriately Tense	(4)Inappropriately Tense
Area 3 = other	(1)Disengaged	(2)Engaged	(3)Appropriately Tense	(4)Inappropriately Tense

4

Communication and Team Skills			
Element	Observed, Adequate	Observed, Mediocre	Expected/Not Observed
Briefing / Re-briefing (formal)			
Verbal Knowledge Sharing - Ideas, Plans, Concerns			
SBAR			
Closed Loop			
Appropriate Conflict Resolution and Assertion			
Debriefing			

5

Threats to Outcome Assessment			
	Not Applicable	Appropriate	Inadequate - Please comment below
Physical environment supports staff			
Equipment and materials support procedures			
Staffing level supports safe care			
Shared mental model is maintained			
Situational awareness is maintained			
Interruptions/distractions are effectively managed			
Clinical support available when needed			
Communication with other departments is coordinated			
Handoffs are comprehensive			
If crisis, **Event manager established**			
Has anyone in the room worked more than 16 hours?		Unknown Yes	

6

Comments

Fig. 1. Front of data sheet. ASA, American Society of Anesthesiologists; BP, blood pressure; HR, heart rate; Intra op, intraoperative; MAP, mean arterial pressure; O₂ SAT, oxygen saturation level; SBAR, situation, background, assessment, and recommendation. (*From* Nurok M, Lipsitz S, Satwicz P, et al. A novel method for reproducibly measuring the effects of interventions to improve emotional climate, indices of team skills and communication, and threat to patient outcome in a high-volume thoracic surgery center. Arch Surg 2010;145(5):489–95; with permission.)

challenges of systematizing observational research techniques and the low incidence of catastrophic failures leading to adverse events. Various approaches have been used to make qualitative research more systematic[9]; however, it remains difficult to control for intraobserver and interobserver assessments of

Definitions of Behavior Markers for CATS Assessment

Climate Score:
Disengaged - Staff in room seem bored, inattentive, distracted
Engaged - Staff seem alert, interested and engaged - appropriate for patient's acuity
Appropriately Tense - Staff seem tense but it is appropriate for what is happening in the case
Inappropriately Tense - Staff seem inappropriately anxious or tense

Briefing/Re-briefing (formal)
   Goals: (Must accomplish both for "Expected and Observed")
     1. Create a shared mental model by discussing pertinent clinical information and an anticipated plan
       of action
     2. Set the tone for collaboration and info sharing by creating and atmosphere of safety to speak up
Re-Briefing (A shortened briefing that occurs if there is a significant change in team members or significant change in the procedure)

SBAR
     Situation
     Background
     Assessment
     Recommendation
Closed loop communication
     Speaking back a teammate's request
     Confirms that the request was heard correctly
     and is being acted upon
     Includes any verbal response including instrument requests met with a verbal response
     Helps the team to maintain a shared mental model.

De-briefing
  Expected during closing segment of case - for scoring purposes only score Adequate or Mediocre if De-briefing occurs during a different segment of case
     Team members are informally assembled after a procedure or activity
       Discuss relevant information for the purpose
         Identifying:
           What went well
           What could have been done differently
           What was learned

Verbal Knowledge Sharing - Ideas, Plans, Concerns
     Any verbal knowledge sharing which is audible to the team or work group and helps to maintain situational awareness and a shared mental model - may include teaching

Appropriate Conflict Resolution and Assertion
     Appropriate assertion of ideas or concerns
     Appropriate negotiation of issues
     Appropriate escalation of concerns including requesting external consultation

Fig. 2. Back of data sheet. ASA, American Society of Anesthesiologists; BP, blood pressure; HR, heart rate; Intra op, intraoperative; MAP, mean arterial pressure; O_2 SAT, oxygen saturation level; SBAR, situation, background, assessment, and recommendation. (*From* Nurok M, Lipsitz S, Satwicz P, et al. A novel method for reproducibly measuring the effects of interventions to improve emotional climate, indices of team skills and communication, and threat to patient outcome in a high-volume thoracic surgery center. Arch Surg 2010;145(5):489–95; with permission.)

behavior and for changes in the subject's behavior simply as a result of being observed, the so-called Hawthorne effect.[10] It is also critical when performing observational research to focus on observed behavior or actions without imputing meaning. Observational research should seek to describe what the subjects are doing (their actions) without speculation regarding reasons, motivations, causes, or effects of behavior.

Another challenge in performing this work is that observers' ability to notice or perceive action or behavior depends on their familiarity with the domain in which they are working. Teamwork research by its very nature involves multiple interactions between subjects of different status with varying role responsibilities. Even when research is restricted to one segment of teamwork, there are still multiple interactions that occur between members in that segment. Domain experts may notice different behaviors than nonexperts, potentially leading to interobserver variation. In addition, intraobserver variation potentially confounds study results when observers do not consistently notice and record similar behaviors at different study periods. These phenomena are not entirely consistent but remain a concern in behavioral research.[11,12]

An additional challenge is that observers tend to focus their attention on areas in which there is the most action, whereas areas of work in which there is less action may equally contribute to outcomes, and these environments are often understudied. Similarly, observers often focus on high-status team members, thereby underobserving the actions of low-status members and the effects that their behavior may have on outcome. Techniques that have been used by research groups to overcome these challenges include formal training of observers using live and/or videotaped interactions, use of multiple observers at one time, routine use of tests of agreement, assessment of interrater and intrarater reliabilities at various phases of a study, and use of standardized observation forms.[12–14]

The Hawthorne effect refers to changes in the subjects' behavior when they know that they are being observed. Techniques to mitigate the Hawthorne effect include having a period of desensitization during which observations are made but data do not contribute to the study. Another approach is to train and use domain-expert observers with whom subjects are familiar. Finally, when teamwork is videotaped, subjects tend to become less sensitized to the fact that they are being observed. Amongst qualitative research experts, although the Hawthorne effect can never be excluded, its effect on research is generally thought to be overstated, as indeed it seems to have been in the work from which the effect took its name.[10]

A final challenge results from the changing configuration of perioperative teams. One approach that has been used by the authors to address this problem is to restrict studies to discrete teams that routinely work together.[5,6,9,15]

Outcome measures

Relating studies of teamwork and communication to discrete outcomes is challenging because most of the outcomes of interest (morbidity, mortality, and serious adverse events) are rare in frequency. Less-rare events, however, such as errors that are compensated, avoiding negative consequences, are less clearly linked to these outcomes of interest. For example, Weinger and colleagues[16] estimated that 27% of anesthetic cases contained a nonroutine event, 17% of which affected the patient and 7% of which resulted in harm. Even such events, however, are difficult to capture, given their unexpected and nonroutine nature. This difficulty makes identifying events of interest that affect outcome onerous and increases the necessary observation time. As a result, adequately powering teamwork and communication studies aimed at outcomes is challenging.

When nonroutine events do occur, actions to address them take place quickly, and it may be difficult for observers to correctly and adequately capture elements of teamwork and behavior preceding, during, and after the event. One solution to this problem is video recording. This approach may allow researchers to retrospectively and robustly analyze teamwork and behavior with respect to discrete events. Another approach used by the authors is to focus on high-acuity cases that routinely involve perturbations in physiology, which if inappropriately managed may lead to catastrophic consequences.[5,6,9,15]

Simulation versus observation

There is significant literature on teamwork and communication based on simulated perioperative environments, however, it is unclear the extent to which data obtained or skills learned in simulated settings are relevant to the actual perioperative environment.[17] Amongst the many challenges of applying research from simulated environments to actual practice is that it is unclear to what extent actors, during simulation, suspend belief. Data on teamwork and communication from simulated environments have, however, been successfully used to generate hypothesis for testing in live environments using observational techniques.[9,18]

Regulatory challenges

There are multiple regulatory challenges to performing observational research.[19] These challenges exist with respect to administrative responses, legal concerns, and human subjects' research oversight in regard to consent and confidentiality. Hospital administrators may be reluctant to permit teamwork research focused on outcomes because of the potential for observational research to highlight and/or document noncompliance with protocols, poor teamwork, and/or poor outcomes.[19] Representatives from specialties being observed, including nursing, may have concerns that observations or study data will be used against individual staff or a particular group of staff. One manner of addressing this concern is to reassure administrators that teamwork and communication research is focused on interactions and not on individual members of the team.

Concern may be expressed that if an adverse outcome occurs during the study, observations from research may be discoverable and weaken the defendants' case because of the documentation of behaviors that could have contributed to the outcome. This concern may be addressed in part by avoiding identifying any individual but instead describing roles (eg, attending surgeon, attending anesthesiologist). In cases in which analysis is possible without roles, they should be omitted. Using standardized observation sheets may also mitigate this risk. Where video recording has occurred, some centers have routinely destroyed footage several weeks after recording, allowing sufficient time to analyze and code data, yet insufficient time for discovery to occur.[19] In addition, researchers can obtain a National Institutes of Health Certificate of Confidentiality. These certificates prevent identifiable research from forced disclosure and are used in situations in which it is difficult to completely protect the identity of subjects.

Teamwork and communication research is subject to the same human subjects research requirements as any other investigation; however, there are several unique challenges with respect to consent and confidentiality (which have already been discussed). The philosophic approach to consent for teamwork and communications research is no different to any other type of study and should seek to inform subjects (physicians, nurses, other operating rooms staff, and patients) of the risks, benefits, and alternatives to participating.

The authors' groups has found that it is instrumental to involve all staff being studied in the design of the study with a view to ensuring that the study aims to address questions that research subjects find meaningful. Leadership from surgery, anesthesiology, and nursing should be engaged early during study design, along with hospital administrators. Once the key research questions have been identified and the study preliminarily designed, information sessions should be held with the subjects to discuss the study and its design, leaving time to enumerate their concerns. Researchers should attempt to address issues that are raised and modify the research plan accordingly before returning to subjects with a finalized research plan.

Subjects should be reassured that their participation in research is purely voluntary and that they can opt out of the research without fear of adverse consequences. When subjects opt in, there is less concern about coercion. Two of the authors of this article used a previously unreported approach in which once 70% of the eligible subjects from surgery, anesthesia, and nursing had opted in for a study, it was authorized to begin.[9] From that point forward, the remaining subjects were only able to opt out. A decision by a subject to opt out must, however, be kept strictly confidential and be made available to the minimum number of investigators and administrators to ensure that the particular subject is not involved in research. It may be useful to provide a contact number to the local human subjects research board, should any subject have concerns that he or she wishes to discuss regarding the study.

In cases in which a patient may be identified in research or the research involves an intervention that may affect the patient, the patient too must provide consent to participate. Patients may need to be reassured that research will not interfere with their routine clinical care.

In addition to these precautions, routine data security precautions should be used, including encoding data and ensuring that data are kept in a password-protected file or a locked room to which only authorized research personnel have access.

SUMMARY

There is a small but growing body of literature demonstrating a relationship between teamwork and communication in the perioperative environment and discrete, measurable, clinically relevant outcomes. Future work in this field should seek to identify which elements of teamwork and communication are most important to improving and/or sustaining good outcomes and preventing the poor ones. Where possible, researchers should seek to use reproducible methods and use standardized data collection instruments.

Although challenging, research should focus on outcomes that are of most value and/or concern to patients, including mortality, morbidity, errors, and other serious adverse events. As an interim step, it may be necessary to focus on proxy measures for these outcomes.

REFERENCES

1. Davenport DL, Henderson WG, Mosca CL, et al. Risk-adjusted morbidity in teaching hospitals correlates with reported levels of communication and collaboration on surgical teams but not with scale measures of teamwork climate, safety climate, or working conditions. J Am Coll Surg 2007;205(6):778–84.
2. Mazzocco K, Petitti DB, Fong KT, et al. Surgical team behaviors and patient outcomes. Am J Surg 2009;197(5):678–85.
3. Nielsen PE, Goldman MB, Mann S, et al. Effects of teamwork training on adverse outcomes and process of care in labor and delivery: a randomized controlled trial. Obstet Gynecol 2007;109(1):48–55.
4. Catchpole K, Mishra A, Handa A, et al. Teamwork and error in the operating room: analysis of skills and roles. Ann Surg 2008;247(4):699–706.

5. El Bardissi AW, Wiegmann DA, Henrickson S, et al. Identifying methods to improve heart surgery: an operative approach and strategy for implementation on an organizational level. Eur J Cardiothorac Surg 2008;34(5):1027–33.
6. Wiegmann DA, ElBardissi AW, Dearani JA, et al. Disruptions in surgical flow and their relationship to surgical errors: an exploratory investigation. Surgery 2007; 142(5):658–65.
7. Lingard L, Espin S, Whyte S, et al. Communication failures in the operating room: an observational classification of recurrent types and effects. Qual Saf Health Care 2004;13(5):330–4.
8. Nurok M, Lipsitz S, Satwicz P, et al. A novel method for reproducibly measuring the effects of interventions to improve emotional climate, indices of team skills and communication, and threat to patient outcome in a high-volume thoracic surgery center. Arch Surg 2010;145(5):489–95.
9. Corbin JM, Strauss AC. Basics of qualitative research. 2nd edition. Thousand Oakes (CA): Sage; 1998.
10. Adair G. The Hawthorne effect. J Appl Psychol 1984;69(2):334–45.
11. Sevdalis N, Lyons M, Healey AN, et al. Observational teamwork assessment for surgery: construct validation with expert versus novice raters. Ann Surg 2009; 249(6):1047–51.
12. Slagle J, Weinger MB, Dinh MT, et al. Assessment of the intrarater and interrater reliability of an established clinical task analysis methodology. Anesthesiology 2002;vol. 96:1129–39.
13. Carthey J. The role of structured observational research in healthcare. Qual Saf Health Care 2003;12(Suppl 2):ii13–6.
14. Weinger MB, Gonzales DC, Slagle J, et al. Video capture of clinical care to enhance patient safety. Qual Saf Health Care 2004;13:136–44.
15. Wiegmann D, Suther T, Neal J, et al. A human factors analysis of cardiopulmonary bypass machines. J Extra Corpor Technol 2009;41(2):57–63.
16. Weinger MB, Slagle J, Jain S, et al. Retrospective data collection and analytical techniques for patient safety studies. J Biomed Inform 2003;36:106–19.
17. Hunt EA, Shilkofski NA, Stavroudis TA, et al. Simulation: translation to improved team performance. Anesthesiol Clin 2007;25:301–19.
18. Bowles S, Ursin H, Picano J. Aircrew perceived stress: examining crew performance, crew position and captains personality. Aviat Space Environ Med 2000; 71:1093–7.
19. Guerlain S, Turrentine B, Adams R, et al. Using video data for the analysis and training of medical personnel. Cogn Technol Work 2004;6:131–8.

Simulation and Quality Improvement in Anesthesiology

Christine S. Park, MD

KEYWORDS

• Simulation • Quality improvement • Translational
• Assessment • Latent condition • Maintenance of certification

Simulation is a systematic approach to ensuring quality and safety of care with the dual benefit of being safe for not only the patient but also the clinician. As a strategy for training, discovering errors and testing solutions, simulation provides an experiential environment in which clinicians may discuss and learn from events that are unconnected to actual adverse events. As such, simulation has become an increasingly widespread approach to provide deliberate[1] and reflective[2] practice and to fill gaps in experience as well as augment overall experience for students, trainees, and practicing clinicians. Furthermore, as graduate medical education faces stricter duty-hour limits to reduce the effects of fatigue on medical error and patient safety,[3] alternate efficacious methods must be found to provide the necessary scope of experience for trainees.

There are about 60 to 70 high-fidelity anesthesia simulation centers to provide education for medical students and trainees throughout the United States. The American College of Surgeons has designated approximately 40 worldwide institutes as level I comprehensive Accredited Education Institutes. Each of these institutes has advanced simulation technology and a focus on surgical trainees.[4] The American Society of Anesthesiologists supports a national endorsement program for simulation centers to ensure that practicing anesthesiologists can also benefit from the advantages of experiential education for the sake of patient safety.[5] With the introduction of simulation as a mandatory component for the American Board of Anesthesiology (ABA)'s Maintenance of Certification in Anesthesiology (MOCA) program, simulation is now formally incorporated into the world of continuing professional practice requirements for board-certified anesthesiologists.[6]

Quality assurance may be defined as "the formal and systematic monitoring and reviewing of medical care delivery and outcome; designing activities to improve

Department of Anesthesiology, Northwestern University Feinberg School of Medicine, 251 East Huron Street, F5-704, Chicago, IL 60611, USA
E-mail address: christinepark@northwestern.edu

Anesthesiology Clin 29 (2011) 13–28
doi:10.1016/j.anclin.2010.11.010   **anesthesiology.theclinics.com**
1932-2275/11/$ – see front matter © 2011 Elsevier Inc. All rights reserved.

healthcare and to overcome identified deficiencies in providers, facilities or support systems; and the carrying out of follow-up steps or procedures to ensure that actions have been effective."[7] The ultimate goal of simulation is to effect results in quality assurance, particularly with respect to the design of activities to improve health care and to overcome deficiencies. How simulation programs affect quality improvement can be analyzed using a translational science framework comprising 3 phases of bench-to-bedside research.[8,9] This article discusses examples of simulation-based research, with a focus on anesthesiology, at 3 different levels using a translational model: (1) as measured in the simulation laboratory, (2) as measured in clinical performance, and (3) as measured in patient outcomes.

TRANSLATIONAL RESEARCH

Translational research refers to a 3-phase process that describes the translation of basic science discoveries into patient outcomes.[10] Phase 1 (T1) begins in the laboratory to bring potential treatments to clinical trial. Phase 2 (T2) examines how the findings from clinical trials apply to actual practice. Phase 3 (T3) incorporates the treatments and strategies, whose efficacies have been demonstrated in Phase 2, into system-wide distillation and sustainable solutions.[11]

Similarly, the conceptual framework for translational research may be applied to examining the effect of simulation for quality improvement. Quality is typically measured in the clinical setting and does not involve a laboratory phase. However, before any simulation-based quality improvement intervention can be introduced in the market, training curricula, or the treatment, can be designed and tested in the simulation laboratory at a T1 level. The primary outcomes are educational outcomes and pertain to the in vitro performance of the clinician, such as improved knowledge, skills, and/or behaviors, as observed in the laboratory setting.

T2 quality improvement using simulation involves the extension of the performance achieved in the laboratory to patient care practices in the clinical setting. The primary outcomes, still pertaining to the performance of the clinician, now feature in vivo demonstration of skills transfer from the simulation laboratory to observed clinical practice.

T3 quality improvement addresses the most challenging and ultimate goal: the extension of clinician performance to accomplish improvement in clinical outcomes. At the T3 level, outcomes pertain to measurable results in patients, populations, organizations, and systems.

HISTORY OF SIMULATORS AND FEATURES OF HIGH-FIDELITY SIMULATION

A simulator is a generic term referring to a physical object, device, situation, or environment by which a task or a series of tasks can be realistically and dynamically represented.[12,13] Simulation is a process or event; it can be defined as "a person, device, or set of conditions which attempts to present evaluation problems authentically. The student or trainee is required to respond to the problems as he or she would under natural circumstances. Frequently the trainee receives performance feedback as if he or she were in the real situation."[14]

Simulation has a long history of use in education and assessment in other high-hazard industries, including aviation,[15] space exploration, war games, and nuclear power plants. In medicine, obstetric mannequin torsos dating to the seventeenth century are among the earliest known simulators.[16] The first reported computer-driven full-body patient simulator was SimOne, developed by Denson and Abrahamson[17] in the 1960s. This mannequin, which could simulate fasciculations to the administration of succinylcholine and seemingly cough in reaction to the presence of the endotracheal tube, faded into obscurity. Two decades later, with the advent of improved computer technology, a full-body mannequin simulator was developed by Gaba and DeAnda[18] as an educational methodology[19] and in the adaption of crew resource management (CRM) to anesthesia crisis resource management (ACRM).[20]

As Edward O. Wilson has stated: "We are drowning in information, while starving for wisdom. The world henceforth will be run by synthesizers, people able to put together the right information at the right time, think critically about it, and make important choices wisely."[21] A simulation platform offers the potential to train and assess such synthetic and dynamic thinking in anesthesiology, as well as a variety of technical and nontechnical skills.

Whether for individual or team performance, technical or nontechnical skills, or novice or expert clinician, high-fidelity simulation is a technology that must be accompanied by certain key features and conditions to facilitate optimal experiential learning and outcomes. These features include providing simulator validity, feedback, repetitive practice, curriculum integration, range of difficulty, multiple learning strategies, a controlled environment, individualized learning, capturing clinical variation, and defining outcomes.[22]

T1 QUALITY IMPROVEMENT: EDUCATIONAL OUTCOMES
Outcome Measures

Individual performance
The preponderance of simulation-based research in medicine is at the T1 level, where educational outcome is the measure. In 1969, Abrahamson, who developed SimOne, was one of the first to comment on educational outcomes for clinical training using high-fidelity simulation. In an experiment training anesthesiology residents in intubation techniques, he observed that residents could achieve proficiency in fewer days of training and this proficiency was achieved in fewer trials in the operating room after having trained on the mannequin, thus contributing to both operational benefit and patient safety.[23] Although the small number of subjects contributed to a lack of significance in most of the analyses performed, more than 40 years later, his concluding recommendation is still current: "the use of simulation devices should be considered in planning for future education and training not only in medicine but in other health care professions as well."

Simulation for T1 quality improvement is not limited to critical events; however, most studies focus on acute-care management scenarios, perhaps because it is during these events that differences in performance could carry the most direct consequences for the patient and provider. Steadman and colleagues[24] studied a group of medical students to compare simulation-based training with problem-based learning. They showed that simulation-based training was a better technique for the acquisition of critical assessment and management skills. An important early milestone for anesthesiology residents is the transition from fully supervised to semi-independent practice, when novice residents must be able to safely provide initial management of a variety of critical events. Park and colleagues[25] studied the efficacy of a simulation-based critical events curriculum for novice anesthesiology residents during their initial weeks of training. In this prospective, observational, crossover study, residents underwent 24 hours of focused simulation-based training for 6 weeks. Trainees were evaluated by blinded raters and demonstrated accelerated acquisition of skills in the management of critical events involving hypoxemia and hypotension. Traditional methods, including didactics and routine clinical operating room care, seemed to be insufficient. The crossover design demonstrated that after training in 1 event, performance was retained during the second 3 weeks while training in the other event occurred.

Johnson and colleagues[26] performed a study for 12 months comparing 2 training methods to teach first-year anesthesiology resident management of adverse airway and respiratory events. The control group was trained using didactics with simulation training, and the experimental group was trained using part-task and variable priority training with simulation. Trainees in the experimental group were able to complete 9% more tasks. Both groups showed an improvement in diagnostic accuracy from 35% to 39% correct to 61% to 73% correct. The investigators showed that the incorporation of additional modes of training could be an effective adjunct to didactic and simulation-based training.

Airway management, especially difficult airway management, is an essential procedural skill for anesthesiologists, yet there are surprisingly little data in the anesthesiology literature investigating simulation-based airway training programs. Goldmann and Steinfeldt[27] studied basic fiberoptic intubation skills in anesthesiology trainees who were trained using an adult virtual reality simulator in addition to didactics and mannequin simulation instruction. After training with the virtual reality simulator, novice trainees significantly improved their time to intubation in a fresh human cadaver,which was not significantly different from that of the attending anesthesiologists. Using a medium-fidelity mannequin simulator, Kuduvalli and colleagues[28] examined the effect of the difficult airway algorithm and technical training for experienced anesthesiologists. The investigators observed that there was a more structured approach for the "can*not* intubate, can*not* ventilate" scenario and an increased use of laryngeal mask airways for the "can*not* intubate, *can* ventilate" scenario. In both scenarios, the incidence of equipment misuse decreased.

Team performance

Teamwork is a complex set of human interactions that has been the subject of extensive research. In 1999, the Institute of Medicine issued a report that specifically identified the promotion of effective team functioning as 1 of its 5 principles to create safe hospital systems.[29] A recent review analyzed those studies seeking T1-type quality improvement outcomes by using "a focus on how to improve (and not only measure) team effectiveness" as an inclusion criterion. The investigators identified several gaps in the literature, including the study of interventions to improve teamwork, the lack of studies in long-term care, and the need for more cohesion and rigorous development of objective outcome measures.[30] Of the studies meeting the inclusion criteria, most studies using simulation training for teams were emergency or trauma teams. Reported quantitative outcomes included improvement in elements of task achievement as measured by timed elements and task completion rates.[30–33] Studies reporting qualitative outcomes were more common, such as changes in attitude and perception about team behavior, communication, and safety climate.[30,34,35]

Mixed findings have been reported on the effect of simulation on teamwork. In a study on simulation by Blum and colleagues[36] that included anesthesiology trainees participating in a 1-day ACRM[20] course, no improvement in team performance in a T1 setting was found. The investigators developed a technique of placing information probes with team members as a means of measuring team information sharing. Using these probes, no change in group sharing was observed from the beginning to end of training. In Sweden, Wallin and colleagues[37] used simulation-based emergency team training for medical students. The investigators observed that despite improvement in team skills, no change in the students' attitudes toward teamwork was registered.

Although this observation is disappointing, one should interpret the results in the context of a reality well recognized by the Federal Aviation Administration (FAA).

The FAA provides a set of specifications on the conduct of CRM training, which has a significant focus on communication and other nontechnical skills. This set of specifications comprises 3 distinct phases: (1) an awareness phase, (2) a skills practice and reinforcement phase, and (3) a continual reinforcement phase.[38] It asserts that "individuals may accept, in principle, abstract ideas, but may find it difficult to translate them into behavior on-the-job." Certain skills, such as communication skills, may have different threshold requirements of the critical element of repetitive practice for learning and for retention.

Impact of Feedback

Providing feedback, or debriefing, is a vital component of any simulation intervention, or indeed any educational intervention, and involves a process of explanation, analysis, and synthesis,[2] with an active facilitator-participant interface. Morgan and colleagues[39] showed that practicing anesthesiologists who received a debriefing after a simulated event demonstrated superior performance by both checklist-based and global ratings compared with those that completed a home study or received no feedback. Savoldelli and colleagues[40] studied the efficacy of 2 types of feedback, oral in-person feedback and video-assisted oral feedback, against a third control group that received no debriefing. There was no difference between the 2 debriefing groups; both groups exhibited improvement in nontechnical skills, whereas the control group did not show improvement. Zausig and colleagues[41] also compared different types of debriefing: a single extensive debriefing encompassing both nontechnical skills and medical management with a simpler medical management debriefing. The group receiving nontechnical skills and medical management debriefing did not prove superior to the group receiving medical management debriefing only. The investigators concluded that a single debriefing may have been insufficient to improve nontechnical skills. By contrast, Yee and colleagues[42] noted an improvement in the nontechnical skills of a group of anesthesiology trainees from the first to second debriefing session but not from the second to third. This range of results may illustrate another layer of need within simulation, that of further inspecting the debriefing process itself.

Assessment Strategies and Tools

As the demand for measures of performance beyond knowledge grows, so does the importance of meeting the challenges of "ensuring that the training program worked."[43] Superior performance assessment design requires a clear definition of skills to be assessed as well as the intended purpose, rigorous construction, and reliability and validity measurements of the test to be used.[44,45] It must also account for issues pertinent to the test subjects, such as level of training or type of practice, as well as the raters, such as conduction of rater training.[45,46]

Several studies elucidate the ability of simulation-based assessments to distinguish performance at different levels of training,[47–50] particularly when a multiple-scenario approach is used,[51,52] thus demonstrating construct validity. Gaba and colleagues[53] have described the features of technical versus nontechnical ratings, while also reporting a large interrater reliability in both technical and behavioral assessment of attending anesthesiologist performance. To capture a broader spectrum of performance, the Anaesthetists Non-Technical Skills behavioral marker system was developed by Fletcher and colleagues,[54] which has been used to assess T1-level outcomes.[42]

A spectrum of scoring tools has been studied, ranging from measurement of timed elements to identification of key actions to rating based on checklists and global measures.[46,51,55–62] Prior work by Hodges and colleagues[63] suggests that global evaluations may be preferable for capturing increasing levels of expertise, whereas checklists may be better suited for novices and may be tailored to the level of training of the participants. Because checklists may provide a more objective means of evaluating observable tasks, interrater reliability has been shown to be higher for checklists than for global ratings.[64] In addition, global ratings, by their very nature, allow for "gestalt" and therefore are also more vulnerable to rater bias. Murray and colleagues[51] evaluated 3 scoring methods: key actions, checklists, and global scores in a simulation-based performance assessment of residents. They observed a high correlation among all the scoring systems and concluded that all scoring systems measured similar performance domains.

To optimize performance assessment tools, one must include other considerations that could confound apparent outcomes. One such consideration is whether performance in 1 critical event scenario can be generalized to performance in other scenarios. As Murray and colleagues[52] report, performance in 1 scenario does not in fact predict performance in other scenarios, thereby suggesting that a given testing event should contain multiple scenarios to obtain a representative sampling of performance.

Another issue of generalization is whether or not performance in critical event scenarios would correlate with that of routine-care scenarios. Critical event management cannot be assumed to be an extension of routine event management by virtue of higher acuity. Although good critical event performance might subsume good routine performance, comparative data are needed. As a start, Zausig and colleagues[65] compared simulation with questionnaires to evaluate the implementation of standard operating procedures for rapid sequence intubation and found that simulation was a useful adjunct to detecting errors in the setting of routine care.

Devitt and colleagues[62] have reported the unexpected finding that university-based anesthesiologists and residents scored significantly higher in a simulation-based assessment than either community-based anesthesiologists or medical students. Because all groups reported that the simulation environment was realistic, familiarity or comfort with the simulation environment was thought to have little effect on the observed performance discrepancy. Such a finding carries far-reaching implications for the assessment of practicing clinicians. It raises critical questions of what aspects of performance merit standardization, what spectrum of performance can qualify as competent, and whether existing performance assessment tools contain too much inherent bias to be applied across various practice settings.

T2 QUALITY IMPROVEMENT: SKILLS TRANSFER

As with any clinically therapeutic intervention, however intuitively appealing the benefits of simulation may be, meaningful outcomes must still be demonstrated. Although lectures and written tests have been vetted for the delivery and assessment of knowledge, competent clinical performance comprises more than knowledge, and research at the T2 level seeks evidence for progression from the simulation laboratory to clinical performance outcomes. McClintock and Gravlee[66] of the ABA noted that in addition to predictors of high performance on the ABA certification examination, "it would be helpful to identify factors that predict clinical performance as well."

The literature contains an abundance of self-efficacy and self-reported attitude data; the simulation literature documents evidence of skills transfer for surgical techniques such as suturing or laparoscopy[67] and improved performance in advanced cardiac life support algorithms.[68,69] However, there are limited data in anesthesiology to show the transfer of simulation-based training to observed clinical practice.

A case report illustrates a T2 (and T3) outcome: a patient receiving a regional block with bupivacaine suffered a cardiac arrest. Two of the anesthesia providers had recently participated in simulation-based training in local anesthetic toxicity. They immediately recognized the presumed cause of the arrest, administered Intra-lipid, and successfully resuscitated the patient.[70] This case exemplifies the goal of most simulation-based interventions for anesthesiology: effective preparation for acute, low-frequency, high-consequence events. Furthermore, it exemplifies a barrier to demonstrating clinical performance outcomes in this and similar settings; the unpredictable occurrence and rarity of real incidents makes many studies simply unfeasible.

When assessing teamwork as the outcome of interest, demonstrating T2 outcomes involves the same challenges as for T1 outcomes. Shapiro and colleagues[71] studied a group of emergency department staff who received an 8-hour intensive simulation training course in addition to a didactic Emergency Team Coordination Course (ETCC). The comparison group was ETCC trained, but instead of simulation, worked together in the emergency department for 8 hours. Teamwork ratings were collected in the emergency department. Although the simulation-trained team showed a trend toward improvement in teamwork ratings after the intervention, differences in performance did not achieve significance in either group.[72]

Bruppacher and colleagues[73] performed a study comparing 2 targeted methods of instruction for weaning from cardiopulmonary bypass (CPB). In this landmark study, which is the first reported randomized controlled trial measuring T2 outcomes for simulation, the investigators studied a group of senior anesthesiology trainees inexperienced in CPB weaning. Trainees received a focused training session in the form of either a high-fidelity simulation or an interactive seminar. The simulation group scored significantly higher than the seminar group in a blinded clinical observation of CPB weaning on 2 testing occasions. Furthermore, it reported the transfer of both technical and nontechnical skills to the clinical setting, thus contributing an important building block in the progress of simulation-based quality improvement in anesthesiology.

T3 QUALITY IMPROVEMENT: CLINICAL OUTCOMES
Can the Effect of Simulation for Quality and Safety Be Measured by Clinical Outcomes?

Demonstrating measurable outcomes for simulation-based quality interventions at the level of populations, organizations, and systems, especially quality and safety outcomes, is the highest level of translational science outcomes. There are several details to be contemplated in this endeavor. First, the terms safety and quality have overlapping domains but are not interchangeable. "'Patient safety' is the avoidance, prevention and amelioration of adverse outcomes of injures stemming from the process of healthcare." On the other hand, "'quality of care' is the extent to which health services for individuals and populations increase the likelihood of desired health outcomes."[74]

Secondly, quality and safety in anesthesia is often monitored by analyzing perioperative morbidity and mortality,[75] but this approach has limited sensitivity and specificity for quality and safety issues. As a result, the anesthesia care task force assembled by the Joint Commission developed anesthesia-related clinical indicators to monitor organizational performance.[76] However, these clinical indicators, comprising sentinel event indicators and rate-based indicators, were developed based on low-level (4–5) scientific evidence in most cases.[77] Given that further development and validation is required for existing clinical indicators, anchoring simulation-based quality improvement to clinical indicators is a considerable challenge.

Finally, there is continuing debate over whether to measure processes versus outcomes. It is easier to address clinician accountability for process measures compared with outcomes, which can be affected by other variables.[78] Furthermore, an outcome such as morbidity and mortality may be an inevitable consequence despite perfect processes, and outcomes may seem unaffected despite flawed processes. Further study will elucidate which process and outcome measures are best influenced by simulation intervention.

T3 Outcomes

Despite the complexities and challenges, evidence exists to support the capacity of simulation interventions to effect T3 outcomes.

In the United Kingdom, neonatal outcomes in deliveries with shoulder dystocia were analyzed before and after the introduction of simulation-based training for the management of shoulder dystocia.[79] A T1 outcome showing improved performance in simulated settings[80] and retention of skills at 6 and 12 months after training[81] had previously been established. Improved clinical performance was achieved in 6 performance variables, thus demonstrating T2 outcomes.[79] Although the rate of shoulder dystocia before and after the training was similar, the incidence of neonatal brachial plexus injury dropped significantly.[78] This result describes a progression of T1 and T2 outcomes to the level of T3 outcomes, resulting from a simulation-based quality improvement intervention.

In another study by Draycott and colleagues,[82] 5-minute Apgar scores and rates of hypoxic-ischemic encephalopathy (HIE) were reviewed before and after the introduction of a 1-day Obstetrics Emergency Training course, which included simulation drills and detailed debriefings for a range of obstetric emergencies. Rates of infants born with low 5-minute Apgar scores as well as infants who developed HIE dropped by nearly 50% in the postsimulation period.

A catheter-related bloodstream infection is an adverse event that is classified by the Center for Medicare Medicaid Services as a nonreimbursable "never event."[83] Barsuk and colleagues[84] created a training module that combined videotaped lecture and simulation curriculum for central venous catheter insertion for trainees. The investigators reported significantly fewer catheter-related bloodstream infections in the period after introduction of the training module than in the period before, during which a series of lectures on bedside procedures was given. Although it is not known whether an alternate method of instruction for central venous catheter placement could have achieved similar results or the videotaped lecture alone would have been sufficient, it is an encouraging indication of the potential of simulation to change outcomes for patients, populations, organizations, and systems.

SIMULATION FOR IDENTIFYING LATENT ERRORS

Threats to the quality and safety of patient care may remain hidden until a triggering event exposes the latent condition.[85] Simulation offers opportunities to discover latent conditions and performance gaps that could adversely affect patient care. Despite anesthesiologists being leaders in promoting a systems approach to patient safety, the anesthesiologist's practice still remains that of a "one-man-band," and the ability to multitask is considered an essential skill. However, this may be a point of vulnerability for errors, which could be alleviated by the presence of a trained assistant. Weller and colleagues[86] performed a prospective observational study to compare the effect of the presence of a trained assistant with that of an untrained nurse in the number of errors made. The investigators showed that the number of errors in the trained assistant group was significantly lower than in the nurse group, thus contributing supporting evidence that a system-based intervention, in this case a trained assistant, may be an important safety intervention by helping to unload the cognitive and task-oriented workload of anesthesiology practice.

Lighthall and colleagues[87] studied a series of unannounced simulated cardiac arrests at various locations within a hospital. These in situ simulations revealed 24 hazardous findings that likely would not have been discovered by a pen-and-paper approach to thinking about potential hazards. As a result, the investigators were able to develop corrective plans and test the effectiveness of changes in later exercises. Howard-Quijano and colleagues[88] identified a performance gap in pediatric resuscitation maneuvers despite acceptable knowledge. In this study of anesthesiology residents, correct performance of chest compressions, administration of the correct epinephrine dose, and appropriate consideration of differential diagnosis was observed in a minority of residents.

Continuing on the theme of cardiorespiratory arrest, Waisel and colleagues[89] performed a simulation experiment to study the management of do-not-resuscitate (DNR) orders by practicing anesthesiologists. The investigators discovered significant inadequacies in the reevaluation of DNR orders and concluded that simulation of perioperative DNR orders could be an effective strategy to test the anesthesiologist's actions in the heat of the moment. Because the policies for the management of DNR orders vary among hospitals and a range of opinions exists regarding the recommendations for DNR orders, simulation could be used to both train and measure awareness and compliance with specific policies.

High-fidelity medical simulation lends itself well to the exploration of the human-machine interface and failure modes of technology and equipment. Mudumbai and colleagues[90] designed a scenario to assess anesthesiology residents' use of anesthesia equipment during a crisis involving a pipeline switch of oxygen and nitrous oxide. The investigators noted multiple failures to recognize and execute corrective measures along with several associated human-machine factors.

Blike and colleagues[91] used a simulated event of pediatric sedation to uncover latent conditions. As the investigators assert, sedation care delivery systems cannot be presumed to be safe without data to asses the efficacy of rescue processes during critical events. This study compared participants' rescue performance in a pediatric sedation critical event to the gold standard of a pediatric anesthesiologist. Significant and critical differences were noted in nonanesthesiologist physician performance in quantitative and qualitative measures, including the time to restore oxygenation, ventilation, and circulation; event-detection errors; management errors; and errors of diagnostic decision making. This methodology of provocative testing highlights simulation as a means to objectively measure safety.

Simulation can be used as a preemptive strategy before the deployment of a new technology or a new procedure. Rodriguez-Paz and colleagues[92] used in situ simulation to identify and mitigate hazards before the implementation of a new technique (high-dose-rate intraoperative radiation therapy). This technology requires coordination of many teams. It involves safety considerations for the providers, including anesthesiologists, surgeons, and radiation oncologists, and patients. By simulating the patient care process, they identified and corrected 20 defects before bringing the first patient to the operating room.

SIMULATION FOR MAINTENANCE OF CERTIFICATION IN ANESTHESIOLOGY

The anesthesiologist provides leadership and takes responsibility for the perioperative journey of patients, including preoperative evaluation, intraoperative anesthetic care, and postanesthetic recovery care. The anesthesiologist is also responsible for the decision whether a particular event during the perioperative period is of enough significance to be considered a critical incident.[93] Thus, ensuring competent performance among practicing anesthesiologists is of utmost importance.

Board certification is considered to be the gold standard in assuring that an anesthesiologist has the knowledge and delivers safe, competent, and quality care, and maintenance of certification is intended to assure that anesthesiologists maintain a standard of excellence. The ABA has recently incorporated participation in a simulation course as a requirement for MOCA. Courses are conducted at a simulation center in the American Society of Anesthesiology's Simulation Education Network. As specified by the ABA, the course must contain scenarios that address, in broad terms, management of significant hypoxemia, hemodynamic instability, and teamwork and communication (http://www.asahq.org/SIM/FAQforSEN.pdf).

At best, board certification is a surrogate indicator of the quality and safety of provider care, and validity studies are few.[94] Could simulation indicators be a reliable and valid approach to assuring performance quality? At present, no summative assessment is associated with participation in simulation for MOCA, as explicitly stated by the ABA, although elements of formative assessment and self-reflection are elemental to the debriefings that accompany simulation. The ASA Web site's FAQ states: "There are relatively few learning forms that help anesthesiologists maintain clinical competence in ways that impact patient care…. There is a belief that simulation will be valuable." (http://www.asahq.org/SIM/FAQforSEN.pdf).

However, the best way to define, observe, and measure performance among practicing anesthesiologists remains unproven. An individual's performance is itself not a static state, and "the response to incidents during anesthesia is a complex process that involves multiple levels of cognitive activity and is vulnerable to error regardless of experience."[50,95] A study investigating the use of simulation as an adjunct to oral examination revealed that the modes of evaluation correlated only moderately and performance varied not only by the mode of evaluation but also by scenario, suggesting that the components of variation in observed performance must be carefully scrutinized.[96]

In the absence of a compelling body of evidence for practicing anesthesiologists, the fact that participants are not formally evaluated may be because of the reality that the validity and reliability of performance measures, as well as the relevant pass-fail benchmarks, are not yet ready for high-stakes use for recertification.

The rapid development and acceptance of simulation makes the question not whether, but how, simulation should be used for continuing professional practice assessment. The ABA was the first to mandate participation in simulation for its maintenance of certification program, but the American Board of Medical Specialties has begun to explore the expansion of simulation for maintenance of certification programs for other specialties.

SUMMARY

High-fidelity simulation is gaining widespread acceptance and use in anesthesiology and other medical specialties, including surgery, obstetrics and gynecology, internal medicine, emergency medicine, and pediatrics. Its use for quality improvement in patient care can be analyzed on 3 levels: the effectiveness of the education (T1), how skills are transferred to clinical performance (T2), and the effect on clinical outcomes (T3).

As simulation for high-stakes assessment becomes inevitable, several questions come to light. Some of the critical questions include the following:

1. How do the performance features of anesthesiologists vary across different practice settings?[62]
2. What is the standard for minimum competence?
3. What scenarios would provide sufficient depth and breadth to fairly represent performance?
4. How should performance be assessed?
5. How should "under-the-bar" performance be addressed?[97]
6. What is an acceptable level of standardization for simulation environments and experiences to minimize the influence of environmental factors on performance?[98]

Simulation has demonstrated results as a strategy to improve performance in providers, facilities, or support systems and, to a limited degree, to improve clinical outcomes. In addition, it can be a valuable strategy to elucidate latent conditions, for which simulation interventions can then be designed. Further research is needed to shed light on active questions such as those presented in this article and to further delineate quality improvement outcomes and future research agendas.

ACKNOWLEDGMENTS

The author gratefully acknowledges William C. McGaghie, PhD for his conceptual framework of education and translational research, and for his continued mentorship. McGaghie is the Jacob R. Suker, MD, Professor of Medical Education and Faculty Development in the Augusta Webster Office of Medical Education at Northwestern University, Chicago, Illinois.

REFERENCES

1. McGaghie WC, Issenberg SB, Petrusa ER, et al. Effect of practice on standardised learning outcomes in simulation-based medical education. Med Educ 2006;40(8):792-7.
2. Rudolph JW, Simon R, Rivard P, et al. Debriefing with good judgment: combining rigorous feedback with genuine inquiry. Anesthesiol Clin 2007;25(2):361-76.
3. Cao CG, Weinger MB, Slagle J, et al. Differences in day and night shift clinical performance in anesthesiology. Hum Factors 2008;50(2):276-90.
4. Smythe WR. The future of academic surgery. Acad Med 2010;85(5):768-74.
5. Steadman RH. The American society of anesthesiologists' national endorsement program for simulation centers. J Crit Care 2008;23(2):203-6.
6. Gallagher CJ, Tan JM. The current status of simulation in the maintenance of certification in anesthesia. Int Anesthesiol Clin 2010;48(3):83-99.
7. Cooper JB, Longnecker DE. Safety and quality: the guiding principles of patient-centered care. In: Longnecker DE, Brown D, Newman M, Zapol W, editors. Principles and practice of anesthesiology. 1st edition. New York: McGraw-Hill, Medical Pub. Division; 2007. p. 20-36.
8. Dougherty D, Conway PH. The "3T's" road map to transform US health care: the "how" of high-quality care. JAMA 2008;299(19):2319-21.
9. McGaghie WC. Medical education research as translational science. Sci Transl Med 2010;2(19):19cm8.

10. Fontanarosa PB, DeAngelis CD. Basic science and translational research in JAMA. JAMA 2002;287(13):1728.
11. Woolf SH. The meaning of translational research and why it matters. JAMA 2008; 299(2):211–3.
12. Good ML, Gravenstein JS. Anesthesia simulators and training devices. Int Anesthesiol Clin 1989;27(3):161–8.
13. Cooper JB, Taqueti VR. A brief history of the development of mannequin simulators for clinical education and training. Qual Saf Health Care 2004;13(Suppl 1):i11–8.
14. McGaghie WC. Simulation in professional competence assessment: basic considerations. In: Tekian A, McGuire C, McGaghie WC, editors. Innovative simulation for assessing professional competence. Chicago: Department of Medical Education, University of Illinois at Chicago; 1999. p. 7–22.
15. Helmreich RL. Safety and error management: the role of crew resource management. In: Hayward BJ, Lowe AR, editors. Aviation resource management. Aldershot (UK): Ashgate; 2000. p. 107–19.
16. Buck GH. Development of simulators in medical education. Gesnerus 1991;48(Pt 1): 7–28.
17. Denson JS, Abrahamson S. A computer-controlled patient simulator. JAMA 1969; 208(3):504–8.
18. Gaba DM, DeAnda A. A comprehensive anesthesia simulation environment: recreating the operating room for research and training. Anesthesiology 1988; 69(3):387–94.
19. Gaba DM. Improving anesthesiologists' performance by simulating reality. Anesthesiology 1992;76(4):491–4.
20. Howard SK, Gaba DM, Fish KJ, et al. Anesthesia crisis resource management training: teaching anesthesiologists to handle critical incidents. Aviat Space Environ Med 1992;63(9):763–70.
21. Wilson EO. Consilience: the unity of knowledge. 1st edition. New York: Knopf: Distributed by Random House; 1998.
22. Issenberg SB, McGaghie WC, Petrusa ER, et al. Features and uses of high-fidelity medical simulations that lead to effective learning: a BEME systematic review. Med Teach 2005;27(1):10–28.
23. Abrahamson S, Denson JS, Wolf RM. Effectiveness of a simulator in training anesthesiology residents. J Med Educ 1969;44(6):515–9.
24. Steadman RH, Coates WC, Huang YM, et al. Simulation-based training is superior to problem-based learning for the acquisition of critical assessment and management skills. Crit Care Med 2006;34(1):151–7.
25. Park CS, Rochlen LR, Yaghmour E, et al. Acquisition of critical intraoperative event management skills in novice anesthesiology residents by using high-fidelity simulation-based training. Anesthesiology 2010;112(1):202–11.
26. Johnson KB, Syroid ND, Drews FA, et al. Part task and variable priority training in first-year anesthesia resident education: a combined didactic and simulation-based approach to improve management of adverse airway and respiratory events. Anesthesiology 2008;108(5):831–40.
27. Goldmann K, Steinfeldt T. Acquisition of basic fiberoptic intubation skills with a virtual reality airway simulator. J Clin Anesth 2006;18(3):173–8.
28. Kuduvalli PM, Jervis A, Tighe SQ, et al. Unanticipated difficult airway management in anaesthetised patients: a prospective study of the effect of mannequin training on management strategies and skill retention. Anaesthesia 2008;63(4):364–9.
29. Kohn LT, Corrigan JM, Donaldson MS, editors. To err is human: building a safer health care system. Washington, DC: National Academy Press; 1999.

30. Buljac-Samardzic M, Dekker-van Doorn CM, van Wijngaarden JD, et al. Interventions to improve team effectiveness: a systematic review. Health Policy 2010; 94(3):183–95.

31. DeVita MA, Schaefer J, Lutz J, et al. Improving medical crisis team performance. Crit Care Med 2004;32(Suppl 2):S61–5.

32. DeVita MA, Schaefer J, Lutz J, et al. Improving medical emergency team (MET) performance using a novel curriculum and a computerized human patient simulator. Qual Saf Health Care 2005;14(5):326–31.

33. Hunt EA, Heine M, Hohenhaus SM, et al. Simulated pediatric trauma team management: assessment of an educational intervention. Pediatr Emerg Care 2007;23(11):796–804.

34. Birch L, Jones N, Doyle PM, et al. Obstetric skills drills: evaluation of teaching methods. Nurse Educ Today 2007;27(8):915–22.

35. Crofts JF, Bartlett C, Ellis D, et al. Patient-actor perception of care: a comparison of obstetric emergency training using manikins and patient-actors. Qual Saf Health Care 2008;17(1):20–4.

36. Blum RH, Raemer DB, Carroll JS, et al. A method for measuring the effectiveness of simulation-based team training for improving communication skills. Anesth Analg 2005;100(5):1375–80.

37. Wallin CJ, Meurling L, Hedman L, et al. Target-focused medical emergency team training using a human patient simulator: effects on behaviour and attitude. Med Educ 2007;41(2):173–80.

38. Baker DP, Beaubien JM, Holtzman AK. DoD medical team training programs: an independent case study analysis. Rockville (MD), Falls Church (VA): Agency for Healthcare Research & Quality (AHRQ): Office of the Assistant Secretary of Defense/Health Affairs (TRICARE Management Activity), U.S. Department of Defense; 2006.

39. Morgan PJ, Tarshis J, LeBlanc V, et al. Efficacy of high-fidelity simulation debriefing on the performance of practicing anaesthetists in simulated scenarios. Br J Anaesth 2009;103(4):531–7.

40. Savoldelli GL, Naik VN, Park J, et al. Value of debriefing during simulated crisis management: oral versus video-assisted oral feedback. Anesthesiology 2006; 105(2):279–85.

41. Zausig YA, Grube C, Boeker-Blum T, et al. Inefficacy of simulator-based training on anaesthesiologists' non-technical skills. Acta Anaesthesiol Scand 2009;53(5): 611–9.

42. Yee B, Naik VN, Joo HS, et al. Nontechnical skills in anesthesia crisis management with repeated exposure to simulation-based education. Anesthesiology 2005;103(2):241–8.

43. Salas E, Wilson KA, Burke CS, et al. Using simulation-based training to improve patient safety: what does it take? Jt Comm J Qual Patient Saf 2005;31(7): 363–71.

44. Boulet JR, Murray DJ. Simulation-based assessment in anesthesiology: requirements for practical implementation. Anesthesiology 2010;112(4):1041–52.

45. Edler AA, Fanning RG, Chen MI, et al. Patient simulation: a literary synthesis of assessment tools in anesthesiology. J Educ Eval Health Prof 2009;6:3.

46. Byrne AJ, Greaves JD. Assessment instruments used during anaesthetic simulation: review of published studies. Br J Anaesth 2001;86(3):445–50.

47. Byrne AJ, Jones JG. Responses to simulated anaesthetic emergencies by anaesthetists with different durations of clinical experience. Br J Anaesth 1997;78(5): 553–6.

48. Forrest FC, Taylor MA, Postlethwaite K, et al. Use of a high-fidelity simulator to develop testing of the technical performance of novice anaesthetists. Br J Anaesth 2002;88(3):338–44.

49. Devitt JH, Kurrek MM, Cohen MM, et al. Testing internal consistency and construct validity during evaluation of performance in a patient simulator. Anesth Analg 1998;86(6):1160–4.

50. Schwid HA, Rooke GA, Carline J, et al. Evaluation of anesthesia residents using mannequin-based simulation: a multiinstitutional study. Anesthesiology 2002; 97(6):1434–44.

51. Murray DJ, Boulet JR, Kras JF, et al. A simulation-based acute skills performance assessment for anesthesia training. Anesth Analg 2005;101(4):1127–34.

52. Murray DJ, Boulet JR, Avidan M, et al. Performance of residents and anesthesiologists in a simulation-based skill assessment. Anesthesiology 2007;107(5):705–13.

53. Gaba DM, Howard SK, Flanagan B, et al. Assessment of clinical performance during simulated crises using both technical and behavioral ratings. Anesthesiology 1998;89(1):8–18.

54. Fletcher G, Flin R, McGeorge P, et al. Anaesthetists' Non-Technical Skills (ANTS): evaluation of a behavioural marker system. Br J Anaesth 2003;90(5):580–8.

55. Morgan PJ, Cleave-Hogg D, DeSousa S, et al. High-fidelity patient simulation: validation of performance checklists. Br J Anaesth 2004;92(3):388–92.

56. Weller JM, Bloch M, Young S, et al. Evaluation of high fidelity patient simulator in assessment of performance of anaesthetists. Br J Anaesth 2003;90(1):43–7.

57. Ringsted C, Ostergaard D, Ravn L, et al. A feasibility study comparing checklists and global rating forms to assess resident performance in clinical skills. Med Teach 2003;25(6):654–8.

58. Boulet JR, Murray D, Kras J, et al. Reliability and validity of a simulation-based acute care skills assessment for medical students and residents. Anesthesiology 2003;99(6):1270–80.

59. Murray D, Boulet J, Ziv A, et al. An acute care skills evaluation for graduating medical students: a pilot study using clinical simulation. Med Educ 2002;36(9): 833–41.

60. Murray DJ, Boulet JR, Kras JF, et al. Acute care skills in anesthesia practice: a simulation-based resident performance assessment. Anesthesiology 2004; 101(5):1084–95.

61. Devitt JH, Kurrek MM, Cohen MM, et al. Testing the raters: inter-rater reliability of standardized anaesthesia simulator performance. Can J Anaesth 1997;44(9): 924–8.

62. Devitt JH, Kurrek MM, Cohen MM, et al. The validity of performance assessments using simulation. Anesthesiology 2001;95(1):36–42.

63. Hodges B, Regehr G, McNaughton N, et al. OSCE checklists do not capture increasing levels of expertise. Acad Med 1999;74(10):1129–34.

64. Morgan PJ, Cleave-Hogg D, Guest CB. A comparison of global ratings and checklist scores from an undergraduate assessment using an anesthesia simulator. Acad Med 2001;76(10):1053–5.

65. Zausig YA, Bayer Y, Hacke N, et al. Simulation as an additional tool for investigating the performance of standard operating procedures in anaesthesia. Br J Anaesth 2007;99(5):673–8.

66. McClintock JC, Gravlee GP. Predicting success on the certification examinations of the American Board of Anesthesiology. Anesthesiology 2010;112(1):212–9.

67. Sturm LP, Windsor JA, Cosman PH, et al. A systematic review of skills transfer after surgical simulation training. Ann Surg 2008;248(2):166–79.

68. Wayne DB, Didwania A, Feinglass J, et al. Simulation-based education improves quality of care during cardiac arrest team responses at an academic teaching hospital: a case-control study. Chest 2008;133(1):56–61.
69. Edelson DP, Litzinger B, Arora V, et al. Improving in-hospital cardiac arrest process and outcomes with performance debriefing. Arch Intern Med 2008; 168(10):1063–9.
70. Smith HM, Jacob AK, Segura LG, et al. Simulation education in anesthesia training: a case report of successful resuscitation of bupivacaine-induced cardiac arrest linked to recent simulation training. Anesth Analg 2008;106(5):1581–4.
71. Shapiro MJ, Morey JC, Small SD, et al. Simulation based teamwork training for emergency department staff: does it improve clinical team performance when added to an existing didactic teamwork curriculum? Qual Saf Health Care 2004; 13(6):417–21.
72. Morey JC, Simon R, Jay GD, et al. Error reduction and performance improvement in the emergency department through formal teamwork training: evaluation results of the MedTeams project. Health Serv Res 2002;37(6):1553–81.
73. Bruppacher HR, Alam SK, LeBlanc VR, et al. Simulation-based training improves physicians' performance in patient care in high-stakes clinical setting of cardiac surgery. Anesthesiology 2010;112(4):985–92.
74. Pronovost PJ, Thompson DA, Holzmueller CG, et al. Defining and measuring patient safety. Crit Care Clin 2005;21(1):1–19, vii.
75. Lee A, Lum ME. Measuring anaesthetic outcomes. Anaesth Intensive Care 1996; 24(6):685–93.
76. Nadzam DM, Turpin R, Hanold LS, et al. Data-driven performance improvement in health care: the Joint Commission's Indicator Measurement System (IMSystem). Jt Comm J Qual Improv 1993;19(11):492–500.
77. Haller G, Stoelwinder J, Myles PS, et al. Quality and safety indicators in anesthesia: a systematic review. Anesthesiology 2009;110(5):1158–75.
78. Rubin HR, Pronovost P, Diette GB. The advantages and disadvantages of process-based measures of health care quality. Int J Qual Health Care 2001;13(6):469–74.
79. Draycott TJ, Crofts JF, Ash JP, et al. Improving neonatal outcome through practical shoulder dystocia training. Obstet Gynecol 2008;112(1):14–20.
80. Crofts JF, Bartlett C, Ellis D, et al. Training for shoulder dystocia: a trial of simulation using low-fidelity and high-fidelity mannequins. Obstet Gynecol 2006;108(6): 1477–85.
81. Crofts JF, Bartlett C, Ellis D, et al. Management of shoulder dystocia: skill retention 6 and 12 months after training. Obstet Gynecol 2007;110(5):1069–74.
82. Draycott T, Sibanda T, Owen L, et al. Does training in obstetric emergencies improve neonatal outcome? BJOG 2006;113(2):177–82.
83. Lembitz A, Clarke TJ. Clarifying "never events and introducing "always events". Patient Saf Surg 2009;3:26.
84. Barsuk JH, McGaghie WC, Cohen ER, et al. Use of simulation-based mastery learning to improve the quality of central venous catheter placement in a medical intensive care unit. J Hosp Med 2009;4(7):397–403.
85. Gaba DM, Fish KJ, Howard SK. Crisis management in anesthesiology. New York: Churchill Livingstone; 1994.
86. Weller JM, Merry AF, Robinson BJ, et al. The impact of trained assistance on error rates in anaesthesia: a simulation-based randomised controlled trial. Anaesthesia 2009;64(2):126–30.
87. Lighthall GK, Poon T, Harrison TK. Using in situ simulation to improve in-hospital cardiopulmonary resuscitation. Jt Comm J Qual Patient Saf 2010;36(5):209–16.

88. Howard-Quijano KJ, Stiegler MA, Huang YM, et al. Anesthesiology residents' performance of pediatric resuscitation during a simulated hyperkalemic cardiac arrest. Anesthesiology 2010;112(4):993–7.

89. Waisel DB, Simon R, Truog RD, et al. Anesthesiologist management of perioperative do-not-resuscitate orders: a simulation-based experiment. Simul Healthc 2009;4(2):70–6.

90. Mudumbai SC, Fanning R, Howard SK, et al. Use of medical simulation to explore equipment failures and human-machine interactions in anesthesia machine pipeline supply crossover. Anesth Analg 2010;110(5):1292–6.

91. Blike GT, Christoffersen K, Cravero JP, et al. A method for measuring system safety and latent errors associated with pediatric procedural sedation. Anesth Analg 2005;101(1):48–58.

92. Rodriguez-Paz JM, Mark LJ, Herzer KR, et al. A novel process for introducing a new intraoperative program: a multidisciplinary paradigm for mitigating hazards and improving patient safety. Anesth Analg 2009;108(1):202–10.

93. Smith AF, Goodwin D, Mort M, et al. Adverse events in anaesthetic practice: qualitative study of definition, discussion and reporting. Br J Anaesth 2006;96(6):715–21.

94. Silber JH, Kennedy SK, Even-Shoshan O, et al. Anesthesiologist board certification and patient outcomes. Anesthesiology 2002;96(5):1044–52.

95. DeAnda A, Gaba DM. Role of experience in the response to simulated critical incidents. Anesth Analg 1991;72(3):308–15.

96. Savoldelli GL, Naik VN, Joo HS, et al. Evaluation of patient simulator performance as an adjunct to the oral examination for senior anesthesia residents. Anesthesiology 2006;104(3):475–81.

97. DeMaria S Jr, Levine AI, Bryson EO. The use of multi-modality simulation in the retraining of the physician for medical licensure. J Clin Anesth 2010;22(4):294–9.

98. Cumin D, Weller JM, Henderson K, et al. Standards for simulation in anaesthesia: creating confidence in the tools. Br J Anaesth 2010;105(1):45–51.

Using Information Technology to Improve Quality in the OR

Brian Rothman, MD[a,b,]*, Warren S. Sandberg, MD, PhD[b],
Paul St Jacques, MD[b]

KEYWORDS

- Information technology • Decision support
- Augmented vigilance • Transparency

The vigilant qualified anesthesia care provider remains the most important guarantor of quality care in the operating room (OR) suite. Vigilance has been described as "requiring a state of maximal physiologic and psychological readiness to act."[1] Maintaining this psychological readiness to act in response to evolving events requires sustained attention and is composed of alertness, information selection, and conscious effort. The vigilant clinician needs meaningful sensory inputs to provide information for analysis and action. At present, a variety of physiologic monitors provide most of the critical information regarding the anesthetized patient's state.

Despite decades of technological development, monitoring remains an array of low-level information used to enable high-level decision making by the anesthesiologist. Analyses of anesthesia closed claims have helped define pulse oximetry, capnography, blood pressure, and the electrocardiogram (ECG) as the most useful monitors.[2] Anesthesiologists use monitors (and other anesthesia equipment such as anesthesia machines) in their quality armamentarium by attending to the normal output and alarms of these devices. It is up to the provider to decide if these alarms and outputs are accurate, and after this decision, what action should be taken with respect to the patient.

This article summarizes the current state of technology as it pertains to quality in the OR and ties the current state back to its evolutionary pathway as a way of understanding how the current capabilities and their limitations came to pass. The article elucidates how the overlay of information technology (IT) as a wrapper around current monitoring and device technology may provide a significant advancement in the ability

[a] Perioperative Informatics, Vanderbilt University School of Medicine, 1301 Medical Center Drive, 4648 TVC, Nashville, TN 37232, USA
[b] Department of Anesthesiology, Vanderbilt University School of Medicine, 1301 Medical Center Drive, 4648 TVC, Nashville, TN 37232, USA
* Corresponding author. Department of Anesthesiology, Vanderbilt University School of Medicine, 1301 Medical Center Drive, 4648 TVC, Nashville, TN 37232.
E-mail address: brian.rothman@vanderbilt.edu

Anesthesiology Clin 29 (2011) 29–55
doi:10.1016/j.anclin.2010.11.006   **anesthesiology.theclinics.com**
1932-2275/11/$ – see front matter © 2011 Elsevier Inc. All rights reserved.

of anesthesiologists to use technology to improve quality along many axes. The authors posit that IT will enable all the information about patients, perioperative systems, system capacity, and readiness to follow a development trajectory of increasing usefulness, as outlined in the following sections.

At present, most information needed to make decisions in the health care environment is concealed. Clinicians must interview and examine the patient to learn symptoms and signs and must search for data in charts and electronic data systems. Turning this flow of effort around so that information comes to the clinician, as well as processing information to amplify its value is the future pathway of technology development to improve quality in the OR. There are 5 successive concepts involved:

- Making information visible without searching creates a form of transparency in the health care environment. Monitors create transparency about the patient's physiology. However, a physiologic monitor leaves most of the key contextual information required to interpret the data concealed in other information repositories.
- Sending information to where it is needed when it is needed creates augmented vigilance. Alarms on monitors are a designed attempt to create augmented vigilance, but again, they only provide limited insight when used in isolation. Ideally, all meaningful information about the patient can be evaluated against expected norms (or a model of the expected process) and exceptions flagged to a clinician at the point of care, which would be true augmented vigilance.
- Providing augmented vigilance with proper contextual cues requires integration of patient and process data. For example, integrating apnea alarms with knowledge that intubation is under way gives context that allows the alarm priority to be downgraded.
- Providing rule-based or knowledge-based recommendations about how to proceed through the medical and/or operational path defines decision support. Decision support goes beyond bringing attention to information. Decision support further seeks to extend the clinician's knowledge base of optimal actions on data made visible through transparency and augmented vigilance.
- Enabling decision support also enables automated process monitoring and process control. This concept can enforce actions that are known or thought to be always beneficial. Worked examples include prompting clinicians to monitor blood pressure when gaps in measurement are detected during anesthesia.[3]

These key conceptual notions of increasing the value added to clinical and medical process information, transparency, augmented vigilance, integration, decision support, and automated process monitoring and process control, map a pathway forward in using IT to improve quality in the OR (**Table 1**).

CURRENT STATE: LIMITED TRANSPARENCY, SINGLE PARAMETER AUGMENTED VIGILANCE AND NOT MUCH MORE

Generation of actionable information requires the anesthesia provider to interpret data and continuously evaluate whether appropriate care is being provided. Clinicians must assess monitor information to decide whether patient goals are being met, usually invoking additional patient information to provide context. The patient's comorbidities, type of surgery, and current state of care during the surgery are critical pieces of information not provided by present-day monitors. During manual procedures competing for clinicians' attention, monitors can be of limited usefulness. The present-day

Table 1	
Key concepts in technology development to improve quality in the OR	
Transparency	Making information available (to the senses, usually visible) without search
Augmented vigilance	Pushing information to the provider at the point of care; goes beyond transparency to make the information active
Integration	Brings information from multiple modalities together to allow higher level decision making
Decision support	Provides recommendations of one or more possible actions on information made available through augmented vigilance
Automated process monitoring and process control	Elevates the priority of a decision support recommendation to something that should be done unless contraindicated by unique circumstances

monitors trigger alarms based on single parameters and rarely inform the clinician of the parameter's context in relation to other patient status indicators. Ideally, the observed data are delivered at the appropriate level of significance without increased workload or information saturation of the clinician.

The level of clinical vigilance required to perform complex monitoring varies throughout a case. Clinician perception of monitor information is often limited to one sensory channel at a time. The information presented must be compatible with the human sense for which it is intended. Once an input is perceived, there is a time lag between input and performance of a primary task motivated by the monitor input. Primary task performance changes when a secondary task is added. This loading may lead to staring longer at the primary instruments, or load shedding by looking less frequently at the secondary instruments. Also, when these secondary instruments are viewed, the information takes longer to process to high-level data. Experience decreases this loading effect.[4] Another determining factor is which senses are being used and how heavily. Having vision already taxed, delivering information through another sense, such as hearing, may be more effective.[5] This concept is the impetus behind providing different monitor modalities in the OR.

Monitor Development, Graphical, Numerical, and Waveform Displays

Early studies show that data from analog displays are easier to process than those from digital displays; however, the use of color on the digital displays improves search time, improving the provider's ability to distinguish critical information from less important data.[1] Rate-of-change displays have also been used to improve response times. Colors are now commonly used to aid in discriminating various graphical and numerical data on the same monitor. There has been no industry standardization of these colors, and some discrimination may be lost when the same color is used to denote different information on different brands of monitor displays.[6] Finally, monitor observation by providers occupies only 5% of the analyzed time, and the time per view was 1 to 2 seconds each. This at-a-glance monitoring may have an effect on both the physical monitor design and the relative perceived importance of visual versus auditory monitors.[7]

Auditory Display Development, Alerts and Continuous Informing

The limitations of providing monitor input via only one sense have led to efforts to extend perception capacity by harnessing additional senses, mainly hearing, as monitor data conduits. A common example is the pulse tone of the pulse oximeter.

Auditory alerts are useful backups because they can be heard from anywhere in the room (ubiquitous) and staff are unable to eliminate them by turning away their attention (obligatory). A common configuration is to provide continuous background information and significant reminders to the anesthesiologist. Studies on using sound with monitors focus on their ability to alert or alarm instead of inform. Using sound to inform has the potential advantage of reducing visual load and allows for eyes-free monitoring.

Audification is the amplification of an existing otherwise unheard sound, used as a monitor. The esophageal stethoscope is an accessible example of audification. Sonification is the continuous auditory display of otherwise silent data, such as the pulse tone conveying the oxygen saturation as measured by pulse oximetry. Earcons deliver information about a variable status through a discrete short sound or sound pattern.[2] Earcons and sonification are different in that the former are used to provide a higher level of information.[2] In the opinion of the Anesthesia Patient Safety Foundation Summit of 2004, variable-tone pulse oximetry combined with capnography can prevent patient incidents when audible.[8] Earcons have been shown in simulator studies to aid the provider in more rapidly identifying oxygen delivery less than the fraction of inspired oxygen of 21%.[9] The same study also demonstrated that the graphics-only display of capnography failed to aid in more rapidly identifying a change in end-tidal carbon dioxide (CO_2) when only a CO_2 change occurs.[9] Audible (sonified) or heads-up display (HUD)–presented capnography and other vital signs have been suggested as developments to improve responses compared with conventional, visual, video-integrated display monitors.[2]

Besides its widespread use in pulse oximetry, sonification has been used in studies with several other silent variables. Clinicians identified events more rapidly when both visual and sonified displays were used, but the accuracy was better with the visual display.[2] Sonification aids in event identification during time-shared tasks, and time-shared task performance may be improved with auditory monitoring. Auditory monitoring has a distinct benefit when performing perceptual-motor tasks while simultaneously attending to monitoring.[2] Furthermore, in 2008, the study by Sanderson and colleagues[8] showed an event detection improvement when advanced auditory displays (respiratory sonification and blood pressure earcons) were used.

Sonification is not a panacea for increasing the provider's receptive capacity for monitoring. ORs are noisy environments, even without the contribution of more sonified monitors. OR noise may cause an acoustic masking of auditory monitor sounds. Clinician adaptation leading to detection extinction (otherwise known as habituation) can result in detection failures. Attentional blindness with auditory monitors can also occur. Conversely, clinicians relying on continuous sounds may respond more frequently to clinically meaningless stimuli, potentially to the detriment of other more relevant tasks. Because of all these potential issues, visual or other monitor types are still needed as backup.

Auditory monitors contribute to noise in the OR. The potential annoyance to other team members caused by the monitor tones and false-positive alarms can lead to the alarms or tones being turned off. The decision to make the auditory display available to everyone or to only the anesthesiologist through an earpiece might require establishing standards based on the type of monitor. If left to each provider, acceptance by the remainder of the OR staff on a case-by-case basis is unlikely. Other potential disadvantages of using an earpiece include tethering of the anesthesiologist by the earpiece cable (or the fussiness of a wireless connection) and auditory separation from the communication of the rest of the OR team.

Combining display modalities has been suggested to improve the accuracy and speed of event detection.[10] Information loading through different modalities has workload benefits. However, input channels need to be integrated first.[2] Studies have shown that sonification causes the fastest response, followed by visual monitors, and the slowest response is caused by sonification combined with visual monitors.[2] Redundant information delivered by more than one modality may create interference and load shedding. Load shedding results from a secondary task workload causing fewer fixations on secondary displays and greater focus on the primary display. When these secondary displays are viewed, it is for a longer period.[4] Tactile stimuli with vibrating wristbands have recently been tried with success to direct pilots to HUD visual cues to improve event detection.[2]

Advanced Integrated Graphical Displays

Single-sensor single-indicator displays present lower-order data. Ecological, metaphor, configural, and emergent feature graphic displays are newer interface design concepts that attempt to present high-level physiologic interpretations based on a computerized algorithm applied to the collected low-level data.[11] Graphically representing higher order properties facilitates faster event identification and response by as much as 2 to 3 minutes.[8] For example, data combinations of tidal volume and respiratory rate and another combination of 5 hemodynamic parameters both showed benefits.[8] Others have shown better awareness of the patient's state.[8] These results are promising, but these outcomes have only been assessed in simulators.[11]

Higher order interfaces may take longer for users to learn to use and interpret properly and may require more provider time during the case. The benefits of these interfaces have been proved in simulators but not in controlled studies along with time-sharing tasks.[2] The controlled simulator environments have not allowed study of artifact or poor instrumentation on the effectiveness of the interface.[12]

Ecological Interface Design

Ecological interface design (EID) has been used in other industries that have complex social and technical systems. The EID theoretical framework, based on the abstraction hierarchy, is used to design human-computer interfaces that improve problem solving when workers face novel situations. To qualify as a true EID, the interface must follow a "skills, rules, knowledge" taxonomy. The skills and rules are meant to save on cognitive resources of the user while supporting knowledge-based behavior. Knowledge-based behavior is error prone during unfamiliar or unexpected events and requires adaptive problem solving.[13] The goal of this technique is to improve performance in an industry compared with the current state of the art.

Displays have used components of this design concept in simulator testing and in practice. An example of this use was the development of a graphical user interface to aid nurses in ventilator management.[14] While the newly developed circular interface was preferred and aided in the interpretation of parameter changes, it performed more poorly at providing an overall patient status and error rate detection.[14]

EID has provided the greatest benefits to less experienced users in other health care settings.[13] EID has not been fully implemented and studied in a clinical setting. It is a new technology that has been primarily focused on the visual perception channel. Currently, EID is more an art than a science, and it is costly to create and study. There are also concerns about how sensor noise (eg, motion artifact in pulse oximetry or electrocautery in ECG) will be handled by such a new more complex system in environments in which sensor failures would worsen performance. Finally, a coordinated integrated system design is required for EID implementation, and this has not been empirically studied.[13]

Getting Information to the Eye: HUD or Head-Mounted Displays

The design of HUDs either projects data on a display in the preferred line of sight (ie, on the wind screen in aviation or automobiles) or via head-mounted displays (HMDs). In anesthesia, all current HUDs use HMD delivery, so the terms are used interchangeably. HMDs deliver information to the user directly and eliminate their ability to remove or have the monitor removed from their line of sight. Essentially, HMD converts the directional optional graphical monitor into a ubiquitous obligatory monitor like the auditory monitors and alerts. These types of displays can be a combination of monocular or binocular and opaque or transparent. Effective spatial information presentation has been shown in aviation, but effective abstract anesthesia data presentation has not been proven.

Some small studies have shown benefits from using HUD. The time to seek graphical data is reduced with HUDs, and use in a simulator showed that providers looked at the patient 48% more, spent 29% less time performing tasks, looked at the regular monitor 89% less, and had 54% fewer attention switches.[2] Users agreed that performing operative tasks was easier and clinical decision confidence was higher. Other studies demonstrate value during busy portions of cases and reduction of the time required for critical event recognition by one-third.[2] The use of HUD while performing intensive primary tasks, such as transesophageal ECG, in the OR has improved primary monitor observation.[15] Whereas some studies have shown that HUDs improve event detection and resolve attention conflicts, others have shown no improvement. At present, the benefits of HUDs are equivocal.[2,8,16]

HMD devices present computer-generated imagery that is superimposed over the wearer's field of view through a head-worn display. The physical design of HMDs can be limiting. Tolerance of the fit, weight, and restriction of head motion and peripheral vision by anesthesia providers is not universal. Transparent monocles with binocular viewing on dynamic backgrounds delay detection times, whereas opaque monocles eliminate depth-of-field viewing.

Aviation studies show that although the HMD data are presented, attention may not be paid to them.[2] This selective attention is especially true during periods of high workload. Cognitive tunneling, the tendency of observers to focus their attention on one area of information while excluding other information presented outside of the area of primary focus, can also occur. Users focus on one particular aspect and do not see the others. Cognitive tunneling is also referred to as inattentional blindness.

Sanderson and colleagues[8] used combinations of advanced auditory displays, HMD, and visual monitors in studies of event detection. They found that auditory display use increased event detection. No improvement was found when an HMD was added to either visual or advanced auditory monitors, or when all the 3 were used in combination.[8] The effectiveness of the various displays seems to be an area of continued research, especially as HMD technology improves and should become better tolerated.

Virtual Reality

Virtual Reality (VR) uses software and hardware to involve a user in an interactive environment that provides haptic cues or kinesthetic feedback. Kinesthesia, the awareness of the relative position and movement of body parts, and haptic cues, including the sense of touch and object firmness or weight, complete the interactive experience when combined with the visual and auditory input channels.[17] Although not necessarily applicable to clinical environments, VR does have the potential to provide robust simulator environments to perform procedure training, practice responses to critical events, and serve as a telepresence to remote locations. Technology advances continue, and it is still hoped that the future will bring this method of training to anesthesiology.[17] Conceivably, VR could also be used to test the efficacy and safety of monitor designs before their physical construction for actual simulator testing and eventual clinical trials.

Anesthesiologist as Integrator: Challenges to the Anesthesiologist's Attention

Vision sense is the key input for establishing transparency about the patient's physiologic well-being in the OR. To overcome the limitations of using just one sensory modality, audification has been added for some monitor modalities and considered for others. However, these efforts still come up against distraction as a potential limiter of performance and hence quality.

Noise levels in the OR can be equal to or exceed that of a freeway. Radios are frequently cited as a source of distraction. However, studies have shown that vigilance can be improved with the addition of music.[8,10] A diverse genre selection is best, and improved performance may depend on the time of day and the type of tasks to be performed. Overall, music has been shown to enhance attention to OR tasks,[8] especially identifying trend judgments.[10]

Computers are another potential distraction. They are ubiquitous in many OR settings, useful for documentation and medical record information retrieval, and provide access to other activities. In locations that provide unrestricted access, users could potentially access shopping sites, social networking sites, multiplayer games, email, and other non–patient-centered activities. Although appearing unprofessional, these activities are not thought to have any effect on patient care. A recent study has shown that anesthesia providers who read intraoperatively do so during low-workload periods (maintenance) and not during induction or emergence. The providers' vigilance was not affected, but the performance of manual tasks, record keeping, and speaking with others decreased.[18] Although computer activities were not specifically addressed, computer use was observed and included in this study as reading. The investigators proposed that combating boredom (resulting from information underload and understimulation) during anesthesia maintenance periods by performing secondary tasks may improve vigilance.[18]

Monitor Development

Devices collecting physiologic information have evolved substantially over many years of gradual development. Interfaces and usability have been the key areas of improvement, driven by the results of multiple human factors studies.[1] More importantly, the methods of message delivery to the clinician have been the subject of scientific inquiry in attempts to increase the amount of information that can be delivered because overloading of a provider's visual modality or introducing a time-shared task can lead to distraction. Auditory monitors can help maintain patient status awareness in these instances. To date, graphic, auditory, and tactile deliveries (as well as combinations of these 3 modalities) have been studied. In addition, the design of visual information presentation is itself a subject of development, seeking to process information to increase its informational value before visual presentation or to allow presentation without requiring the anesthesiologist to look away from the patient. These developments can be conceptualized as attempts to improve the transparency of physiologic information and to create augmented vigilance. However, definitive proof that there is an improvement in patient outcome from enhanced monitors remains elusive. Moreover, there is little progress toward integrating information from other domains. Hence, decision support, such as it is, addresses only the narrow silo of physiologic data.

GETTING FROM PATCHY TRANSPARENCY TO INTEGRATED DECISION SUPPORT

The economics of anesthesiology suggest that workload will increase over time. Thus, anesthesiologists will be under increasing pressure to adopt technology that allows them to focus more on high value-adding tasks.[19] Activities such as solution preparation[20] and visual collection of data for manual recording and integration are obvious targets to go by the wayside. Time-motion studies, although flawed, provide us with the best information about the complexities of performing a safe anesthesia procedure. Recommendations, even 10 to 15 years ago, from these studies suggest the benefit of automated record keeping and integrated monitoring and alarms.[1]

Monitoring is in development to improve local transparency about the physiologic state of the patient but still does not provide higher order data about patient medical status or data about operational and system status. Developing monitoring to acquire such data is the next frontier of research and development aimed at making anesthesiologists more productive while improving the quality of the work they do.

Improvements from Current Technology

The individual workplace, the single OR, where one spends an entire workday with one patient at a time is becoming obsolete. Anesthesiologists move between care locations, are responsible for multiple patients at once, and are increasingly appreciating the effect of single-OR decisions on the function of the entire perioperative system.[21–23]

Creating transparency must go beyond the single OR to encompass all the necessary perioperative system. Data delivery to providers outside the OR has also developed over the last few decades. Beginning in 1994, the Vanderbilt Perioperative Information Management System (VPIMS) documentation suite has provided an example of a perioperative information management system (PIMS) that aggregates data from multiple sources for integrated display. VPIMS represents a concerted effort to provide transparency about medical and process-of-care trajectories to clinicians and managers throughout the perioperative environment. Specifically, the Vigilance system (Acuitec LLC, Birmingham, AL, USA), a component of VPIMS developed at the Vanderbilt University School of Medicine, integrates and aggregates data from numerous clinical monitors and hospital information systems. Aggregated data are transparently provided to all appropriate staff throughout the perioperative process in real-time. Consistent with its design, the VPIMS also provides interfaces allowing admitting, nursing, and anesthesia staff to update the system with real-time data that are automatically synchronized and disseminated throughout the perioperative arena. This process yields improved transparency about patient status (**Fig. 1**). Intuitively, this improved transparency should improve patient care, safety and efficiency.

VPIMS interfaces with applications such as OR scheduling, electronic health record (EHR), patient location, billing, computerized physician order entry, and web-based alphanumeric paging. Integrated synchronized patient data are used by authorized users based on their role. As the patient is cared for in the preoperative, intraoperative, and postoperative settings, medical record documentation is entered and collected through desktop or laptop computers at each point-of-care location and stored on a central server. This thin-client methodology keeps sensitive patient health information from being stored on point-of-care devices. Desktop computers with a keyboard and mouse or trackball is the most common hardware configuration in the OR, and each is associated with (and transmits data from) a physiologic monitor.

Real-time OR admission, discharge, and transfer (ADT) information is transparently displayed on case boards mounted at strategic locations across all perioperative care areas. The graphical displays also present additional ADT information via color codes and icons. These graphical displays provide more detailed data regarding key perioperative status changes, thus providing transparency of data to assist floor managers and clinical personnel with OR workflow management and planning. Icons may be assigned to cases to assist with patient and staff. Users who have appropriate access can also access case list boards from any institutional computer, either as a stand-alone program or embedded in selected interfaces to support transparency (**Fig. 2**).

This transparency-at-a-glance potentially increases efficiencies and economies in the OR suite on a daily basis.[24] For example, Xiao and Dexter found that people used transparency systems to see if cases were finished, to see if a room was ready, and to see when cases were about to finish. In other words, transparency systems can be used to support workflow decisions.[12] At Vanderbilt, the display of real-time room status through electronic case boards and live room video allow for informed management decisions without having to walk through a 35-room OR suite. The displays may also enable operational efficiency through economies of scale for the perioperative process.

VPIMS is complimented by Vigilance (see **Fig. 1**), an application that provides transparency and augmented vigilance at locations remote from the anesthetizing location via desktop or mobile devices. Situational awareness (SA) programs, such as Vigilance, can be stand-alone programs or be integrated with existing perioperative and hospital systems. Authorized users are presented with live video, graphical vital sign trends, monitor waveforms, EHR, communication, and OR protocols.

A notification engine in Vigilance provides, for the first time, augmented vigilance for both patient data and system status data. Specifically, Vigilance informs users of out-of-range vital signs, administration of certain medications (eg, vasopressors), as well as changes in patient location or OR turnover status. Users subscribe to notifications for ORs and patients for whom they are caring. Notifications are processed through central stations and received by subscribers through the desktop program, pagers, short message service, and other push notification technologies. Vigilance is used in daily practice and provides augmented vigilance by bringing issues such as critical drug administration and out-of-norm physiology to the attention of decision makers, (who may be physically removed from the OR) at the same time the in-room providers receive the information. "I was about to page you" is a frequent comment from OR anesthetists when these decision makers enter a room in response to a notification.

Access to Vigilance data has important implications for management of large OR suites, if change-in-status data about the medical trajectory of cases are delivered to OR managers. These integrated data are also available via smartphones (ie, iPhone or BlackBerry) and other mobile devices, implying that critical patient information is always available to the clinician. This transition has opened up a new area of research to probe the efficacy of such modalities related to patient care, patient safety, and OR efficiency.

PIMS technology can also aid the team-level SA in the OR. Using a large computer display as a patient-specific and case-specific whiteboard, the entire Vanderbilt OR team reviews and verifies specific critical case information during the hard-stop pre-procedure time-out for each case in every Vanderbilt OR. The surgeon leads the time-out and discusses standard time-out questions with the staff. During this session, the staff verbally verify each item of the time-out checklist as it pertains to the chart documentation, the patient information on the board, and the information physically present on the patient in the room (armband) (**Fig. 3**). During this process, the other staff in the room stop their activities to listen and review the information displayed on the electronic whiteboard, and they either agree or disagree with every step

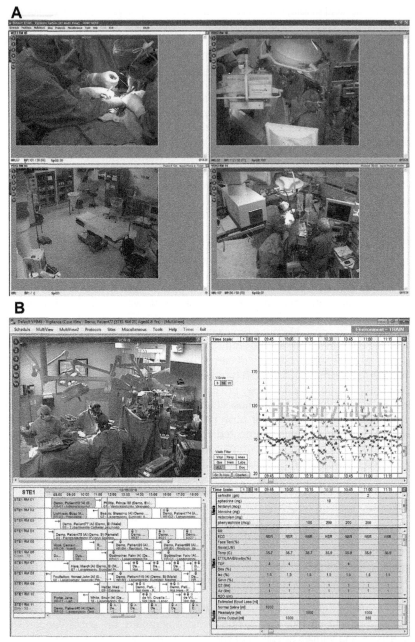

Fig. 1. (*A*) An example of Vigilance live video. Shown is a multiview mode with 4 rooms viewed simultaneously. Each room's most current vital signs are beneath each view and status notifications can be seen in the upper right corners. (*B*) An example of Vigilance integrating data from patient monitors and live video and scheduling data in a single view. (*C*) A view of Vigilance live video combined with real-time monitor waveform visual display. This is half of a 4-quadrant display. (*Courtesy of* Acuitec LLC, Birmingham, AL, USA; with permission.)

C

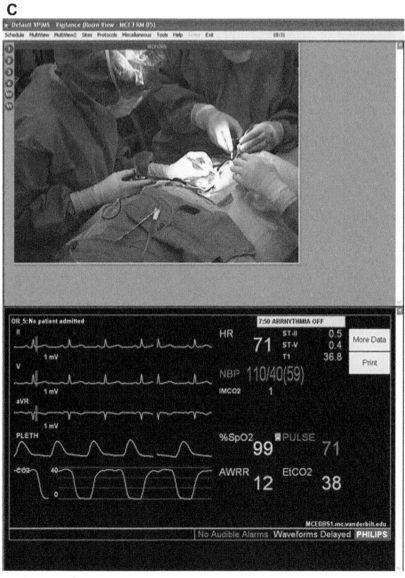

Fig. 1. (*continued*)

of the process. As each step of the time-out is completed, the circulating nurse docu-ments it in VPIMS. Recent VPIMS software developments synchronize data between the whiteboard and the nursing documentation systems. An update is specifically generated from nursing documentation to the electronic whiteboard for each step in the time-out process. Thus, each step is sequentially visually displayed as pending (red) or checked off (green) as the time-out process proceeds (see **Fig. 3**A). Displaying data in this way provides a reproducible scaffold for the activity, makes the time-out transparent, and creates shared awareness of patient data related to the time-out. Any staff present in the room can delay incision if he or she thinks that any portion of the time-out discussion is incorrect. The use of PIMS technology is one of the

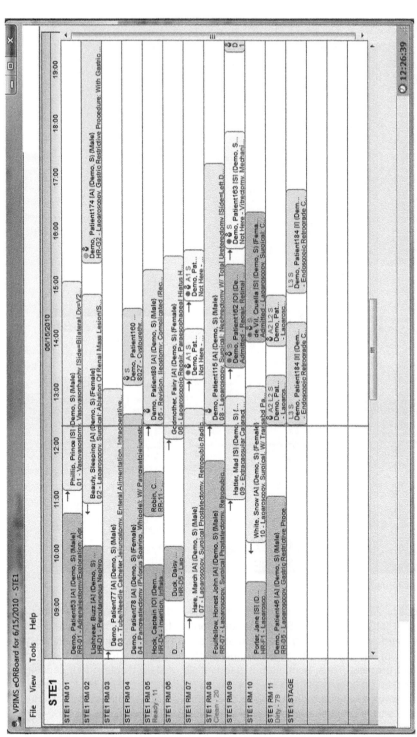

Fig. 2. An electronic schedule board provides access to current scheduling information to perioperative staff. Data presented may include patient-specific and procedure-specific information, information about patient readiness for surgery, information about room setup status, and case start or completion delays. Using this information, managers can project room occupancy and arrange the schedule to maximize efficiency, whereas clinicians can use the same information to obtain critical patient information. (*Courtesy of* Acuitec LLC, Birmingham, AL, USA; with permission.)

A

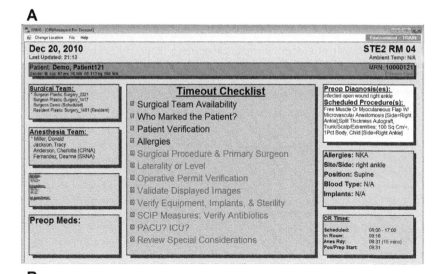

B

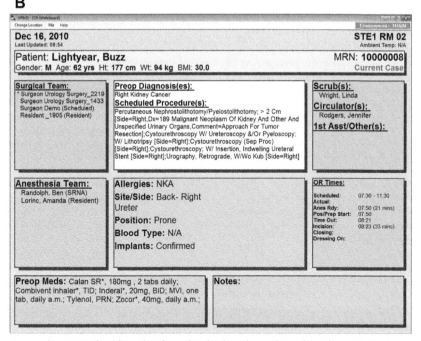

Fig. 3. An electronic checklist whiteboard is displayed on a large liquid crystal display panel in the OR to assist in team SA and safety to perform a preprocedure time-out. (*A*) Example of a preprocedure time-out board during the surgical safety checklist. As each item is documented to be complete, it turns from red to green on the display. (*B*) After checklist completion, the board displays key patient, case, and staff information.

many possible examples of how information systems may improve safety and patient care. Vanderbilt researchers are currently assessing the effect of implementing this visualization system on the before-implementation and after-implementation performance quality of the time-out process.

HOW AUGMENTED VIGILANCE AND DECISION SUPPORT CAN IMPROVE
PROCESS-OF-CARE QUALITY PERFORMANCE

Real-time integration of electronic data allows one to go beyond transparency to provide augmented vigilance and decision support. The process flow diagram of a basic decision support system (DSS) is given in **Fig. 4**. A fundamental requirement for automated DSSs is a process model against which actual process action can be

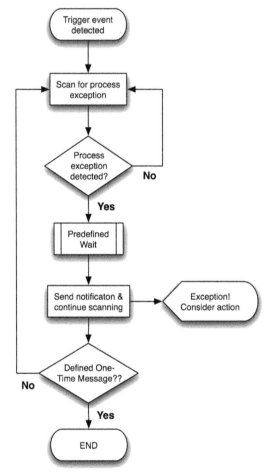

Fig. 4. Generic decision support workflow diagram. "Trigger event" is the event that starts the monitoring algorithm. In anesthesia, this event is frequently something related to the beginning of the case. "Process exception" is a generic term indicating that the monitored process is not progressing according to the process model defined by the user. Process models against which actual process execution can be compared are the key features. Although the process model itself can often be very simple to state (eg, "preoperative anti-biotic management should be documented before incision" or "the patient should go only to their scheduled OR") the underlying logic and database queries that support process monitoring can be quite complex. When a process exception is detected, the system gener-ates a notification (Exception! flag in the figure). Notifications are pushed to the relevant stakeholders to provide the information as soon as it is known, with the goal of providing information when it is most beneficial. In other words, the system ideally provides a reminder just before it is needed.

compared. The process model can be as simple as "event X should occur before event Y."

Some of the best new automated DSSs touch on clinical care by enhancing the execution of specific process-of-care tasks. Notable examples from Vanderbilt relate to execution of perioperative measures from the Surgical Care Improvement Project (SCIP). SCIP is a national quality partnership of organizations focused on improving surgical care by significantly reducing surgical complications. The SCIP goal is to reduce the incidence of surgical complications nationally by 25% by 2010[25] through implementation of a set of evidence-based practices. Many (although not all) of these measures are initiated in the perioperative period. Hence, automation applied through a PIMS can be used to improve performance on those goals that are amenable to automated perioperative data collection.

Prophylactic antibiotic administration within 1 hour before surgical incision and appropriate redosing during long cases is aided by a forced prompt in intraoperative systems, such as those developed by VPIMS, General Electric Centricity, and Massachusetts General Hospital (MGH). MGH and VPIMS prompts are designed to track the documentation of antibiotic decision-making before incision (**Fig. 5**). The options presented as part of the decision-making process include (1) antibiotic administration before incision, (2) antibiotics given on inpatient unit, (3) administration of antibiotics held so that culture material could be obtained, (4) use of antibiotics held at surgeon's request. Taken together, these criteria allow administrators to track perioperative decision making and documentation on antibiotic administration as metrics. The system prompts the user with a default behavior but allows for specific acceptable exceptions to the common practice. Algorithms applied through the MGH system maintained a 98% compliance rate for preincision documentation of antibiotic decision making for years (Stephen Spring, Department of Anesthesia, Critical Care and Pain Medicine, MGH, unpublished results, 2009) and VPIMS has had similar sustained unpublished success.

Initiation of β-blocker therapy (in appropriate patients) to decrease perioperative cardiac ischemic events is another example of a process measure included in SCIP. VPIMS uses the preoperative evaluation, preoperative nursing, and intraoperative anesthesia systems in a conditional forced-function manner to guide the use of

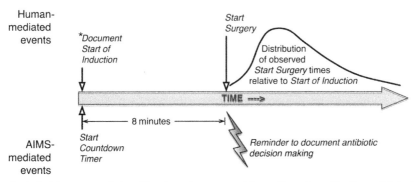

Fig. 5. A decision support algorithm based on a countdown timer from the time of "start of induction". The timer reminds the clinician via an automated prompt to document prophylactic antibiotic decision making before a surgical incision. The 8-minute delay was based on observations of the actual latency between documentation of start of induction and actual surgery start time (defined as incision). The asterisk indicates single checkbox, reliably and contemporaneously entered as part of anesthesia workflow. AIMS: Anesthesia Information Management System.

perioperative β-blocker management according to the SCIP guidelines. The system incorporates data such as whether a patient is on β-blocker therapy, the time and date of their last dose, and the time of incision, and then the anesthesia provider is queried regarding intraoperative administration, providing a reminder to meet the SCIP guideline. Data demonstrate that the local compliance of the system is higher than 90% (Paul St Jacques, Vanderbilt University School of Medicine, unpublished data, 2010).

Normothermia, another SCIP measure, is tracked by VPIMS. Ambient room temperature is measured and added to the medical record so that it can be correlated to patient temperatures perioperatively. These data are currently being collected and will add to the existing knowledge of the effect of room temperature and its direct and indirect effects on postoperative infection. Hair removal using clippers instead of razors and deep vein thrombosis prophylaxis are other SCIP measures for which prompts have been inserted into PIMS to aid in compliance, and more importantly, improve patient care by allowing OR teams to manage toward goals for performance, which can be set in the context of current performance.

PIMS-based decision support tools have also improved compliance with pay-for-performance (P4P) measures. However P4P implementation has not been consistent, and results have varied.[26–30] In one instance, a real-time decision support engine that uses different algorithms to assess records for a variety of potential errors that would interfere with billing has been shown to improve financial performance in the department in which it was developed.[31] This result has important implications, because the same system has been subsequently adapted to decisions affecting clinical quality, with essentially no added cost.[3,32] Hence, the quality enhancement system is commensally connected to a direct revenue stream.

Future State: Workload Distribution and Decision Support Engines

PIMS is increasingly instituted and used for documentation, management, billing, quality of care, and compliance. In addition, management and staff often desire real-time data to make decisions. Although PIMS can be used to accomplish this goal, DSS latency must be considered. DSS latency has been defined as the time between when a DSS query would have triggered an event message and the time of the event itself. Latency is determined by when the event was recorded in the database (not the time of the event itself).[33] Query frequency, missing documentation, and documentation timeliness affect this value. Latencies can be a liability and should be considered in real-time DSSs because large differences in event times and the time the event is recorded in the database could adversely affect clinical and managerial decisions.

One of the uses of PIMS decision support is to facilitate reallocations of resources. Currently, we rely on the individual provider to communicate to others when additional assistance is required, including not only assistance in the OR with a catastrophic event but also assistance with other ORs they may be covering simultaneously, such as when a provider is performing a high-workload task in one of those rooms. Workload distribution can therefore affect the care of individual patients, multiple patients, and OR efficiency and management. Predictive algorithms would ideally account for each patient's stability, comorbidities, surgical procedure complexity, and the intraoperative status. This information would then be combined and applied to the respective providers caring for the patients to determine each supervising provider's workload. Either a user or the system could trigger a reallocation notification when an evolving event is identified. Events may be as benign as 2 rooms ready to start simultaneously or as significant as a cardiac arrest. For the relatively benign managerial decision, Dexter and colleagues[34,35] have provided a framework for day-of-surgery decision making and demonstrated that anesthesiologists benefit from support even for these seemingly straightforward decisions.[36,37]

Notification should reflect the event's significance. For example, managerial decisions have lower priority than medical decisions, especially those known to affect outcome. Depending on the severity and location of the event, future DSSs would use intelligent algorithms and indoor location systems to review the available providers with the appropriate skill set, evaluate their respective workloads and proximity to the event, and assign notifications to each provider based on the proximity and workload. Proof-of-concept using patient locations has demonstrated that indoor location systems can provide the needed personnel location data.[38]

The system would then monitor the responses to the notifications. For example, if a nearby, low-workload responder did not move to the event, their workload should be reassessed to ensure that it has not changed. If there were no change, a follow-up notification would be sent. Simultaneously, the other providers would be tracked. Notification escalation to others including the OR management would be considered if the response to the event was not sufficient.

The obstacles to developing such a system are significant. Inaccurate or incomplete algorithms may cause inaccurate reallocations, false events that waste resources, or worst of all, missed events in which no reallocation occurs. Although event latency has been discussed, this issue will become more significant as more systems are added as real-time interfaces to the decision engine. Asynchronous event documentation or computation is especially problematic. For example, large amounts of discrete and free text medical data entering an engine from multiple software packages could make even the most accurate algorithms flawed. Maintaining such a system will be resource heavy from both computing and personnel perspectives.

More importantly, the issue of asynchronous event entry in anesthesia care must be addressed before medical decision support can be effective. For example, if automatic alerts and prompts are to improve anesthesiologists' selection of drugs, there must be a change in work practice so that the planned administration of drugs is always entered into the system before the event. This entails complete reorganization of one of the most fundamental subroutines of anesthesia workflow – a habit ingrained from an anesthetist's first moments in training and reinforced by decades of repetition. These complex decision engines are likely many years away, but at present, there is technology to begin construction of systems that will serve as a foundation for the future.

MOBILE DEVICES FOR THE MOBILE ANESTHESIOLOGIST

Computer workstations are a staple in many health care settings. These workstations often require providers to leave the bedside to document. Similarly, remotely supervising multiple locations with PIMS or SA systems has traditionally required the use of a fixed desktop personal computer (PC) workstation.[39,40] Such supervision also relies on the care providers in the care locations to notify the supervising physician as events not visible to the computer occur or evolve. Anesthesiologists are rapidly being freed from their desktop workstations by new generations of smartphones. Vanderbilt University Medical Center's iPhone app, VigiVU, works in conjunction with the SA program Vigilance.

VigiVU brings vital sign data to the clinician through a mobile device, enabling proactive decision making. The device also receives live room video, vital signs, and notifications of predetermined out-of-range vital signs. Access to laboratory values and history and physical information is also available (**Fig. 6**). This access

A

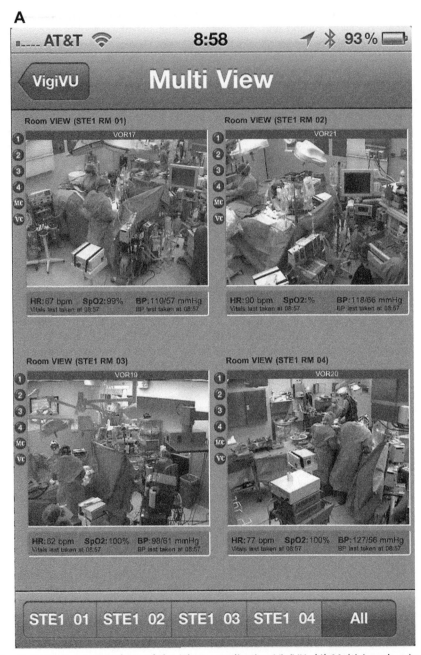

Fig. 6. Case view screen shots of the iPhone application VigiVU: (*A*) Multiview showing 4 rooms simultaneously. (*B*) Communication panel with the room and staff signed into the case. (*C*) Focused history and physical. (*D*) Room video with current vital signs. (*E*) Graphical vital signs trends.

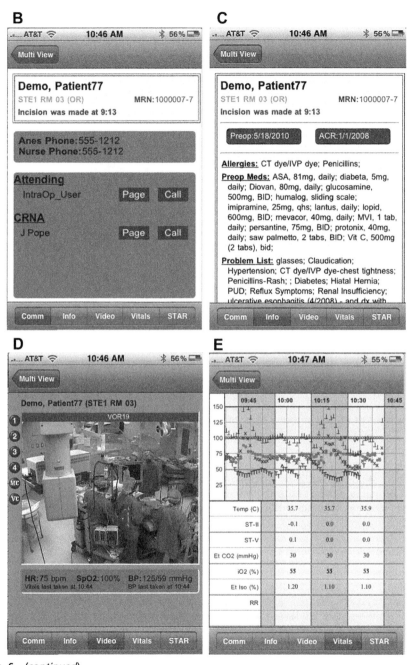

Fig. 6. (*continued*)

allows clinicians to learn of evolving intraoperative events at essentially the same time as in-room staff (**Fig. 7**) and to pull in contextual information from medical history. The mobile devices allow clinicians to directly communicate with room personnel to guide management either from another care area or while traveling to that care location.

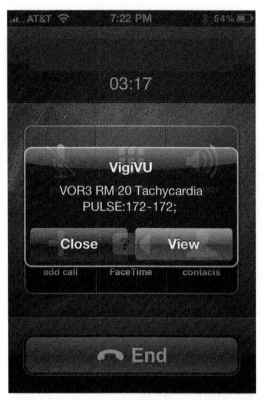

Fig. 7. Out-of-range vital signs. Rooms are subscribed to so that the user can receive push notifications of vital signs that are out of range, as well as conventional pages.

VigiVU also allows providers access to the OR case board with color-coded indicators of patient status and location with an option of detailed and summary views. Anecdotally, OR management and prioritization of secondary care tasks have been made easier using the application (**Fig. 8**). The authors believe that mobile technology can match clinicians' increasingly mobile practice demands.

Technology Considerations: Open versus Closed Platforms

The dominant mobile device software platforms are currently Android, iPhone, WebOS (Palm), RIM (Blackberry), and Windows Mobile. The physical device required for each system, feature variety, platform and application stability, and ability to deploy at the enterprise level vary. When developing new software, the question of whether to use an open less-restrictive or a closed more proprietary platform is a debatable topic. A more open platform can allow for some interesting, creative, and flexible features for users and may be easier to deploy throughout the enterprise.[41] However, some think that this model is chaotic, error prone, and results in low-quality design and features. There can also be a lack of accountability and lack of, or multiple, standards.[41] Closed platforms are often perceived to be draconian in their practices and require approval before features are implemented. Development can be faster and more efficient, however, because there is usually a single format, and operating system patches usually consider compatibility.[41] Closed platforms

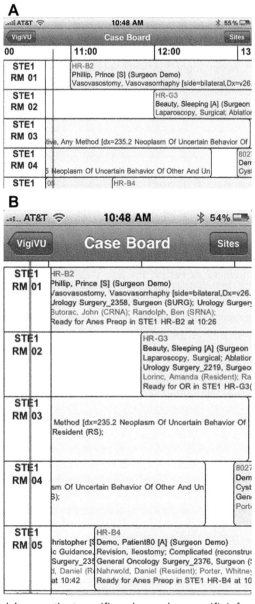

Fig. 8. OR case board shows patient-specific and procedure-specific information, information about patient readiness for surgery, room setup status, and case start or completion delays. Managers can project room occupancy and arrange the schedule to maximize efficiency, and clinicians use the same information to obtain critical patient information. (*A*) Summary view provides basic case information, maximizing the number of cases visible per view. (*B*) Detailed view provides more information on each case, and fewer cases are visible per view.

tend to be superior when dealing with security concerns and system freezes from side-loaded unapproved or unverified applications.

Hardware considerations are equally important. Smaller devices may be convenient, but the reduced screen size presents a glaring limitation with respect to displaying large amounts of information. Users may have difficulty entering information and/or reading from a small screen. Some may prefer using a desktop PC or tablet as their primary resource. To accommodate the variety in preferences, the concept of a single piece of hardware or software in health care being everything to everyone must be abandoned. Accordingly, it is best to make mobile applications run alongside desktop applications rather than replacing desktop applications entirely.

Potential Limitations (Real and Political)

Even today, there is considerable skepticism to overcome about the value of computerizing ORs. One concern about adding computers to the OR (for anesthesia record keeping and nursing perioperative documentation) is that they actually distract the anesthesiologist from patient care. However, concerns about attention and distraction predate computers in the OR. In 1971, an ergonomics study found that 42% of an anesthesiologist's time was not directed at the patient.[1] Since then, manual record keeping has not been shown to alter vigilance.[42] However, there are factors about computerizing the workspace that may affect attention. For example, the location of the computer used for anesthesia data collection is intuitively such a factor.

The computer can either be placed in the line of sight with the patient (on the left side of the anesthesia machine) or behind the anesthesiologist (on the right side of the machine). The effect of computer location on direct patient observation and the receipt of higher-level information is currently unknown. Many currently popular anesthesia machines are designed so that it is almost a requirement to place the computer on the right, essentially enforcing a paradigm wherein anesthesiologists must turn their backs to the patient to document. The authors believe this design is not correct because it requires attention to be diverted from the patient. Moreover, the right-mounted design forces documentation to be discontinuous and retrospective rather than (at least potentially) more continuous and contemporaneous. This form of documentation, in turn, worsens the problem of latency,[33] thus complicating the problem of creating near real-time DSSs.

The integration of live video from the OR into the application enhances transparency. Video provides a significant opportunity to improve the SA of a supervising clinician who cannot always be physically present in the OR. However, video can be difficult to implement in certain environments. Anesthesia providers in the room may feel like someone is always looking over their shoulder. Other staff may have identical concerns compounded by fears of potential medicolegal discovery. Assuring staff that the video is not stored in any way and is for real-time display only has been helpful at Vanderbilt. Also successful, the University of Maryland records video on optical disk that automatically overwrites every 72 hours. The staff has agreed to allow video use for teaching purposes. Either all consent to be shown in the video or identifying features are blurred.[43,44]

Staff may also have a fear regarding the perceived loss of autonomy or of closer performance monitoring. There may be unfounded concerns that the video is going to be recorded for future review or punitive action. Patients may have concerns regarding stored data being misused or mishandled, resulting in the loss of privacy. These issues provide the opportunity for education of patients and staff alike. Lack of user acceptance has led to a 30% failure rate in new applications in other health care domains.[45] Educating staff about the video's intended use in a staged manner improves the chance of acceptance.[45] The technology acceptance model suggests that the perceived ease of use directly affects the perceived usefulness and these together best predict system use.[45] Technical support and training have no effect.[46] Questionable and even inappropriate behaviors can also occur. Clinicians may access the video for cases for which they are not responsible. Others may feel the systems are sufficient for medical supervision and reduce their time in the OR. These behaviors may diminish the benefits of the SA system. User-specific system activity logs to review appropriate versus inappropriate system use may be necessary.

Proving the benefits of the various technologies aiming to create transparency, augmented vigilance, and decision support remains a significant challenge. It has been suggested that measuring the speed and accuracy of emerging event identification, workload reduction, incident management, and overtreatment reduction[2] may be areas in which advantages are seen. With respect to creating transparency about patient physiology, no single monitor to date has demonstrated improved outcomes, including pulse oximetry. The combination of multiple monitors and clinical interpretive skills provide such a high level of safety that any additional benefit from new technology may be difficult to demonstrate. Institutional IT initiatives tied to patient safety initiatives perform better than those that do not use IT solutions.[47] Studies such as that of Toomey and colleagues[48] that have demonstrated that displaying radiological information on mobile devices provides clinicians with important information and may be comparable to viewing images on secondary monitors are a beginning.

Because it is yet to be proved that new technology can improve care and safety should this be used? Smith and Pell[49] question the use of parachutes to prevent major trauma from gravitational challenges. Their point is well made; perhaps not all interventions are suited to the rigors of evidence-based medicine evaluations. The workflow, workload, ocular tracking, event identification, and response studies that have been performed, combined with the observational data will need to suffice until definitive studies can be conceived and performed.

SUMMARY

Future anesthesia care providers will use a combination of auditory and visual tools in the OR that not only alert but also inform. Advanced EID displays with supporting algorithms that promote proactive decision making will inform the provider of potential events through appropriate sensory channels that the system identifies as not overloaded. As the event develops, the system adapts by load shedding inputs to other sensory channels for the provider, diminishes OR noise, eliminates non–patient-centered activities, and adds the current alert to all sensory channels to focus the provider's attention on the predicted event. The monitor information available to the provider will be presented as high-level information that is patient and situation contextual. Suggested courses of action based on best practices are presented, or a specific action will be required if the best practice is unequivocal. The immediate supervising anesthesiologist outside the room is made aware of the predicted event. These anesthesiologists follow the event evolution and observe the same best practice recommendations presented to in-room providers on their mobile device. The earcons and sonifications heard in the room are remotely delivered through an earpiece. Escalation alerts to the surrounding team based on workload, skill set, and need are made accordingly as resources are reallocated to assist. VR, HMD, and HUD interfaces will be available for providers, supervisors, and managers.

Real-time integration of patient information is necessary to make this future a reality. EHR systems have generally mimicked our previous system of hand-written records and allow a great deal of free text entry that is not discrete. This lack of discreteness creates a significant challenge, but reflecting a change in health information from one point of care across an entire system is considered the ideal. The lack of discrete, structured, machine-readable data makes consistent data exchange between systems difficult. Without consistency, algorithms applied to these data may misinterpret or ignore information that is critical to the care of the patient. Either our data will need to become more discrete (and defined) or the decision support engines will need to be extremely adaptive. Otherwise, the information will be without appropriate context.

Automated process monitoring and process control systems must process the context of new information and self-correct. The incorrect addition or deletion of information in this system is immediately propagated throughout the entire system. Imagine a malignant hyperthermia diagnosis entered in error by another service while an anesthetic is being performed. But decision support and process controls should realize that the patient has received a depolarizing agent and anesthetic vapor with no ill effects and not alarm the provider. Resolution of health information conflicts may require users to reevaluate the diagnosis and correct it manually, or could be performed by the system automatically.

There have been great strides to develop and implement technology to provide and improve transparency and augmented vigilance. We have even seen some inroads in integration and decision support. These systems are not yet ubiquitous, however. Adding computers to the OR and providing video for SA has met with some skepticism that should wane as improved outcomes are shown.

The current technology is laying the groundwork to create systems with integration, decision support, and automated process monitoring and process control. As these systems are constructed, it is important to determine whether safety, efficiency, and patient outcomes are improved. This determination should begin by probing the benefits of each individual component and concept as it matures. As integration between the systems evolves, interaction synergies and conflicts will be discovered and will require study and provide improvement opportunities. As the technology leaves the simulators and is delivered to the patients, multicenter collaboration through databases such as Multicenter Perioperative Outcomes Group[50] will be essential to obtain a sufficiently powered study to test whether operational or medical benefits accrue.

When the proposed future state can be achieved is an open question. The computational and cultural hurdles seem daunting. However, recall that the iPhone is less than 3 years old. The pace of platform technology is accelerating, and the technological capability may be just around the corner. The question then becomes whether anesthesiologists are culturally ready for decision support and process monitoring and process control. Harnessing expectations about technology in everyday life (where antilock brakes are a tangible example of automatic process monitoring and process control) may raise expectations and circumvent our resistance to these potentially quality-enabling systems.

REFERENCES

1. Weinger MB, Englund CE. Ergonomic and human factors affecting anesthetic vigilance and monitoring performance in the operating room environment. Anesthesiology 1990;73(5):995–1021.
2. Sanderson PM, Watson M, Russell W. Advanced patient monitoring displays: tools for continuous informing. Anesth Analg 2005;101(1):161–8.
3. Ehrenfeld JM, Epstein RH, Bader S, et al. Automatic notifications mediated by anesthesia information management systems reduce the frequency of prolonged gaps in blood pressure documentation. Anesthesia & Analgesia 2011, in press.
4. Harris RL, Tole JR, Stephens AT, et al. Visual scanning behavior and pilot workload. Aviat Space Environ Med 1982;53:1067–72.
5. Wickens CD. The structure of attentional resources. In: Nickerson RS, editor. Attention and performance VIII. Hillsdale (NJ): Erlbaum; 1980. p. 239–57.

6. Mitchell MM. Human factors in the man-machine interface. In: Gravenstein JS, Newbower RS, Ream AK, et al, editors. The automated anesthesia record and alarm systems. Boston: Butterworths; 1987. p. 33–48.
7. Ford S, Birmingham E, King A, et al. At-a-glance monitoring: covert observations of anesthesiologists in the operating room. Anesth Analg 2010;111(3): 653–8.
8. Sanderson PM, Watson M, Russell W, et al. Advanced auditory displays and head-mounted displays: advantages and disadvantages for monitoring by the distracted anesthesiologist. Anesth Analg 2008;106(6):1787–97.
9. Lampotang S, Gravenstein JS, Euliano TY, et al. Influence of pulse oximetry and capnography on time to diagnosis of critical incidents in anesthesia: a pilot study using a full-scale patient simulator. J Clin Monit Comput 1998;14: 313–21.
10. Sanderson PM, Tosh N, Philp S, et al. The effects of ambient music on simulated anaesthesia monitoring. Anaesthesia 2005;60(11):1073–8.
11. Michels P, Gravenstein D, Westenskow DR. An integrated graphic data display improves detection and identification of critical events during anesthesia. J Clin Monit 1997;13:249–59.
12. Reising DV, Sanderson P. Minimally adequate instrumentation in an ecological interface may compromise failure diagnosis. Hum Factors 2004;46:316–33.
13. Vicente. Ecological interface design: progress and challenges. Hum Factors 2002;44(1):62–78.
14. Liu Y, Osvalder AL. Usability evaluation of a GUI prototype for a ventilator machine. J Clin Monit Comput 2004;18(5–6):365–72.
15. Platt MJ. Heads up display. Br J Anaesth 2004;92(4):602–3.
16. Liu D, Jenkins SA, Sanderson PM, et al. Patient monitoring with head-mounted displays. Curr Opin Anaesthesiol 2009;22(6):796–803.
17. Burt DE. Virtual reality in anaesthesia. Br J Anaesth 1995;75(4):472–80.
18. Slagle JM, Weinger MB. Effects of intraoperative reading on vigilance and workload during anesthesia care in an academic medical center. Anesthesiology 2009;110(2):275–83.
19. Sandberg WS. Barbarians at the gate. Anesth Analg 2009;109(3):695–9.
20. Fraind DB, Slagle JM, Tubbesing VA, et al. Reengineering intravenous drug and fluid administration processes in the operating room: step one: task analysis of existing processes. Anesthesiology 2002;97(1):139–47.
21. Sandberg WS, Canty T, Sokal SM, et al. Financial and operational impact of a direct-from-PACU discharge pathway for laparoscopic cholecystectomy patients. Surgery 2006;140(3):372–8.
22. Sandberg WS, Ganous TJ, Steiner C. Setting a research agenda for perioperative systems design. Semin Laparosc Surg 2003;10(2):57–70.
23. Butterly A, Bittner EA, George E, et al. Postoperative residual curarization from intermediate-acting neuromuscular blocking agents delays recovery room discharge. Br J Anaesth 2010;105(3):304–9.
24. Xiao Y, Hu P, Hu H, et al. An algorithm for processing vital sign monitoring data to remotely identify operating room occupancy in real-time. Anesth Analg 2005; 101(3):823–9.
25. Available at: http://www.qualitynet.org/dcs/ContentServer?c=MQParents&; pagename=Medqic%2FContent%2FParentShellTemplate&cid=1228694349383& parentName=Category. Accessed July 28, 2010.
26. Lin GA, Redberg RF, Anderson HV, et al. Impact of changes in clinical practice guidelines on assessment of quality of care. Med care 2010;48(8):733–8.

27. Alshamsan R, Majeed A, Ashworth M, et al. Impact of pay for performance on inequalities in health care: systematic review. J Health Serv Res Policy 2010; 15(3):178–84.

28. Duszak R, Saunders WM. Medicare's physician quality reporting initiative: incentives, physician work, and perceived impact on patient care. J Am Coll Radiol 2010;7(6):419–24.

29. Hilarion P, Suñol R, Groene O, et al. Making performance indicators work: the experience of using consensus indicators for external assessment of health and social services at regional level in Spain. Health Policy 2009;90(1):94–103.

30. Mehrotra A, Pearson SD, Coltin KL, et al. The response of physician groups to P4P incentives. Am J Manag Care 2007;13(5):249–55.

31. Spring SF, Sandberg WS, Anupama S, et al. Automated documentation error detection and notification improves anesthesia billing performance. Anesthesiology 2007;106:157–63.

32. Sandberg WS, Sandberg EH, Seim AR, et al. Real-time checking of electronic anesthesia records for documentation errors and automatically text messaging clinicians improves quality of documentation. Anesth Analg 2008;106(1): 192–201.

33. Epstein RH, Dexter F, Ehrenfeld JM, et al. Implications of event entry latency on anesthesia information management decision support systems. Anesth Analg 2009;108(3):941–7.

34. Dexter F, Epstein RH, Traub RD, et al. Making management decisions on the day of surgery based on operating room efficiency and patient waiting times. Anesthesiology 2004;101(6):1444–53.

35. McIntosh C, Dexter F, Epstein RH. The impact of service-specific staffing, case scheduling, turnovers, and first-case starts on anesthesia group and operating room productivity: a tutorial using data from an Australian hospital. Anesth Analg 2006;103(6):1499–516.

36. Dexter F, Willemsen-Dunlap A, Lee JD. Operating room managerial decision-making on the day of surgery with and without computer recommendations and status displays. Anesth Analg 2007;105(2):419–29.

37. Dexter F, Lee JD, Dow AJ, et al. A psychological basis for anesthesiologists' operating room managerial decision-making on the day of surgery. Anesth Analg 2007;105(2):430–4.

38. Sandberg WS, Hakkinen M, Egan M, et al. Automatic detection and notification of "wrong patient-wrong location" errors in the operating room. Surg Innov 2005; 12(3):253–60.

39. iMDsoft. Available at: http://www.imd-soft.com/. Accessed July, 2010.

40. VISICU. Available at: http://www.healthcare.philips.com/main/products/patient_monitoring/products/eicu/index.wpd. Accessed July, 2010.

41. Ingram M. Open vs. closed: In the ongoing battle over control, how much is too much? Available at: http://gigaom.com/2010/04/20/open-vs-closed-in-the-ongoing-battle-over-control-how-much-is-too-much/. Accessed July, 2010.

42. Loeb RG. Manual record keeping is not necessary for anesthesia vigilance. J Clin Monit 1995;11(1):9–13.

43. Guzzo JL, Seagull FJ, Bochicchio GV, et al. Mentors decrease compliance with best sterile practices during central line placement in the trauma resuscitation unit. Surg Infect (Larchmt) 2006;7:15–20.

44. Xiao Y, Seagull FJ, Bochicchio GV, et al. Video-based training increases sterile-technique compliance during central venous catheter insertion. Crit Care Med 2007;35:1302–6.

45. Kim YJ, Xiao Y, Hu P, et al. Staff acceptance of video monitoring for coordination: a video system to support perioperative situation awareness. J Clin Nurs 2009; 18(16):2366–71.
46. Wu JH, Wang SC, Lin LM. Mobile computing acceptance factors in the healthcare industry: a structural equation model. Int J Med Inform 2007;76(1):66–77.
47. Menachemi N, Saunders C, Chukmaitov A, et al. Hospital adoption of information technologies and improved patient safety: a study of 98 hospitals in Florida. J Healthc Manag 2007;52(6):398–407.
48. Toomey RJ, Ryan JT, McEntee MF, et al. Diagnostic efficacy of handheld devices for emergency radiologic consultation. AJR Am J Roentgenol 2010;194(2): 469–74.
49. Smith GC, Pell JP. Parachute use to prevent death and major trauma related to gravitational challenge: systematic review of randomised controlled trials. BMJ 2003;327(7429):1459–61.
50. Multicenter Perioperative Outcomes Group. Available at: http://www.mpog.med. umich.edu/. Accessed November 10, 2010.

Using Real-Time Clinical Decision Support to Improve Performance on Perioperative Quality and Process Measures

Anthony Chau, MD[a], Jesse M. Ehrenfeld, MD, MPH[b],*

KEYWORDS

- AIMS • OR • Perioperative quality • Real-time data
- Clinical decision support

OVERVIEW

Anesthesia information management systems (AIMS) are becoming more commonplace in operating rooms (ORs) across the world and have the potential to help clinicians measure and improve perioperative quality. However, to realize the full potential of AIMS, clinicians must first understand their capabilities and limitations. This article reviews the literature on AIMS, focusing on areas where AIMS have been shown to have a meaningful effect on quality, safety, and operational efficiency.

INTRODUCTION TO AIMS
History and Market Penetration

Since the days of Harvey Cushing at the beginning of the twentieth century, the maintenance of an accurate and detailed perioperative patient record has been a foundation for providing safe anesthetic care.[1] Historically, handwritten paper records have been the sole means of documentation during an anesthetic event and are still the method of data collection in many parts of the world. However, monitoring systems in the OR have become progressively more complex, and the amount of real-time physiologic data continues to expand exponentially. In response to this information

Disclosure: There are no relevant financial conflicts to disclose.
a Department of Anesthesiology, Pharmacology and Therapeutics, University of British Columbia, 3200-910 West 10th Avenue, Vancouver, BC V5Z1M9, Canada
b Department of Anesthesiology, Vanderbilt University, 1301 Medical Center Drive, 4648 TVC, Nashville, TN 37232-5614, USA
* Corresponding author.
E-mail address: jesse.ehrenfeld@vanderbilt.edu

overload, new computer systems have been developed to help collect, manage, store, and interpret the exponential amount of data that are now available to clinicians. Now, anesthesia providers worldwide are gradually adopting AIMS to aid with the collection and interpretation of perioperative data through a set of tools collectively known as clinical decision support tools.

Modern-day AIMS are a combination of hardware and software systems designed to facilitate the automatic recording, storage, and retrieval of perioperative data for surgical patients.[2] Although AIMS have been around in various forms for several decades, their widespread adoption has been hindered mostly by financial barriers, complexities of system installation, and a perceived lack of proven benefits.[3] In 2001, no more than 1% of all departments in the United States were using AIMS; five years later, this number had only increased to 5%.[4] However, in 2007 a major paradigm shift began to occur along with the digitization of other parts of most hospitals, such as radiology and pharmacy, and more academic anesthesia departments in the United States were beginning to adopt AIMS.[5] By 2008, at least 14% of the anesthesia departments in United States were using AIMS, and 44% of academic anesthesia departments have adopted or planning to implement an AIMS.[3,6] Outside of the United States, similar trends have been seen in Europe, and a recent survey of European university-affiliated hospitals revealed that 15% of the anesthesia departments had already adopted AIMS.[6]

Core Functionality

Since their inception, AIMS were designed to reliably manage charting duties by accurately capturing intraoperative data and events in real time. Most AIMS allow for both the automatic transcription of data from intraoperative physiologic monitors (eg, vital signs and ventilator settings) and the manual entry of case events (eg, start of surgery, estimated blood loss, and drugs administered) into the electronic record. Critical data elements are often highlighted for the end user to view and, in some cases, respond to through an electronic acknowledgment.

Current systems have expanded their functionality by incorporating preoperative and postoperative information. The more advanced versions are further equipped with clinical decision support capabilities that interact with the end users to facilitate prompt, safe, and accurate decision making. For example, some preoperative evaluation modules provide robust, electronic, history-taking questionnaires and suggest preoperative laboratory tests based on customizable algorithms that take into account the specific procedure and any comorbidities for a particular patient.[3] Complex scoring systems for risk stratifications of patients, such as the European System for Cardiac Operative Risk Evaluation for cardiac surgery, Model for End-stage Liver Disease score for liver resection, or Revised Cardiac Risk Index, can be easily and rapidly calculated using existing laboratory data or via a drop-down menu for quick data entry.[7] AIMS are also capable of rapid integration of internal data with that from external databases. For example, AIMS can facilitate information flow to providers downstream of the OR (ie, recovery rooms and intensive care units) to improve continuity in patient care.

The major advantage of collecting data through AIMS is that the data are consistent, legible, and reliable.[8] Multiple studies have shown that information technology can reduce the frequency of a variety of different types of errors and the frequency of associated adverse events.[8–11] For instance, the dosing of a drug can be accurately calculated using the patient's weight and automatically corrected for renal function. Medications that are infused continuously can be monitored in real time and cross-checked with algorithms that provide real time notifications throughout the perioperative period. **Fig. 1** is a schematic overview of an AIMS that demonstrates how OR physiologic monitors, AIMS workstations, AIMS servers, hospital enterprise-wide clinical information systems, and hospital paging functions can be integrated to provide clinical decision support.

Major Vendors and Systems

High initial capital is typically required to install an AIMS, and cost is by far the single most important factor involved in the purchasing decision. Cost of an AIMS can vary substantially depending on the vendors and systems. Systems may differ in terms of their overall ease of use, functionality, display of and access to intraoperative data, system stability, and security.[3] In 2010, an AIMS workstation and server software alone cost around US $4000 to $9000 per clinical workstation.[12] Additional expenses,

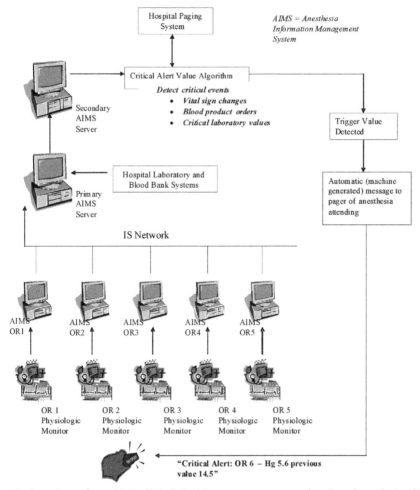

Fig. 1. Overview of an AIMS clinical decision support system showing the relationship between OR physiologic monitors, AIMS workstations, AIMS servers, hospital enterprise-wide clinical systems, and hospital paging functions.

such as software licenses, training and support, maintenance and servicing, warranty and implementation, are further added costs.

AIMS-BASED EVENT REPORTING AND TRACKING TO IMPROVE QUALITY

The ability of an AIMS to accurately and reliably capture intraoperative events is the fundamental strength in which AIMS are able to help clinicians improve quality of anesthesia care. Compared with handwritten records, electronic reports of the time frame of periods of interest (eg, an adverse event such as a cardiac arrest or desaturation) can provide high-resolution details that can help clinicians understand the potential cause of an adverse event and ultimately improve their practice. In addition, AIMS can simplify the process of giving regular feedback to providers regarding their clinical care on an individualized basis.

Improvements in Data Capture and Record Quality

Most investigators would agree that AIMS records are more reliable, less biased, and more accurate than paper records (**Box 1**). In fact, the question of whether it is possible for an anesthesia provider to maintain an accurate intraoperative record while simultaneously exercising clinical vigilance has been challenged by multiple studies. Because the definition of accuracy is not consistent in different studies, it has been difficult to appreciate the true rate of inaccuracy found in written anesthesia records.[13] Despite the discrepancies, most studies conclude that the difference in accuracy and completeness between written and electronic records is most evident during induction and emergency from anesthesia.[14] During these instances, charting has a low priority compared with accomplishing more urgent direct patient-care tasks. In a study of 30 patients undergoing eye surgery, Lerou and colleagues[14] showed that there were many missing and erroneous data in handwritten records during the induction of anesthesia and toward the end of the case. The missing data during those periods seem to be similar, and anesthesiologists did not return to fill in the missing information after the case had concluded.

In more urgent situations, such as during cardiac resuscitation, many rapidly changing physiologic and event data are generated in a short period. Although most code teams assign one individual record data, this rarely happens in the OR during acute situations. However, AIMS are able to markedly enhance the capture of large volumes of data at all points within the perioperative period while the anesthesia provider concentrates on clinical activities.[15] In addition to providing reliable data capture, AIMS-based charting has the further advantage of allowing the clinicians to view the accumulating anesthesia records in real time in a legible and customizable

---

Box 1
Bias, reliability, and accuracy

Bias

Recorder bias is the discrepancy between the expectation of a recorder and the actual (ie, true) value of the parameter being recorded.

Reliability

Reliability is the degree to which a set of measurements is consistent, it is related inversely to random error

Accuracy

Accuracy is the degree of closeness of a set of measurements to its actual (ie, true) value

format that can facilitate the recognition of critical pieces of information that might otherwise remain undiscovered.[16]

Several studies have shown that manually documented anesthesia records often lack sufficient details and valuable information when compared with electronic records.[1,8,14,17] In addition, handwritten records may be biased because of how the anesthesia provider interprets or recalls a situation from memory with a tendency to record data that make sense as opposed to data actually provided by an intraoperative monitor. According to a study by Sanborn and colleagues, only 4.1% of 434 adverse events detected with an AIMS were reported voluntarily.[13] Hollenberg and colleagues[18] compared handwritten anesthesia records with a computerized record during coronary artery bypass surgery and found that significant systematic biases were detected in the blood pressure data in the handwritten records. They found that lower values were recorded as higher values and vice versa. Because of the minimization of the extremes otherwise seen on the computerized record (known as smoothing), the investigators advised that the information from handwritten records lacked accuracy and hence should not be used for research purposes.[18] One center undertook a retrospective study evaluating gaps in vital signs recording. In that study, a series of 200 consecutive handwritten records were found to have no gaps in vital signs recording, whereas an equivalent sample of electronic records from the same time period had gaps in vital signs recording, ranging from 1% to 14% depending on the parameter evaluated and reflecting such periods as when monitors were disconnected to turn a patient to a prone position.[19] This finding is again consistent, with other studies showing that handwritten records are not as accurate as electronic records because of smoothing.[20-22]

Improvements in Adverse Event Tracking

The ability of AIMS to record large volumes of patient and event information with high resolution and fidelity is particularly useful for adverse event investigation and tracking. The ability to use the perioperative data for quality assurance research is enabled and enhanced because the data collected are consistent, reliable, comprehensive, and, most importantly, unbiased.

Rohrig and colleagues[9] performed a retrospective analysis of AIMS data from 58,458 patients undergoing noncardiac surgery. In this study, the investigators detected 17.5% of intraoperative cardiovascular events using AIMS as opposed to the 6% to 15% described in earlier studies using manual recordings.[23-27] The higher incidence of cardiovascular events was most likely secondary to more accurate and automatic record keeping and, hence, more available data for adverse event detection.[9]

Provider-Level Reporting of Quality Measures

Many anesthesia departments are now using AIMS to facilitate the reporting of an increasing number of quality measures that would otherwise be difficult and expensive to perform manually. Because of AIMS ability to store and generate reports electronically, they can also facilitate the dissemination of quality measures at the provider level under many circumstances. This type of individual reporting has been shown in several studies to be a successful technique to encourage providers to improve their performance and change their behavior.[3,16,28,29]

Timely administration of prophylactic antibiotics has been closely examined and used by national quality assurance programs, such as Surgical Care Improvement Project and Agency for Health care Research and Quality, as a quality measure within perioperative medicine.[10] Surgical site infections are a frequent cause of morbidity and mortality and contribute to prolonged length of hospital stay and increased cost of care. It is thought that antibiotic prophylaxis is most effective when administered 30 to 60 minutes before incision. At the University of Michigan Health System, O'Reilly and colleagues[16] found on manual chart review that only 69% of eligible patients received prophylactic antibiotics as per the accepted guideline. Subsequently, the investigators designed a project using an AIMS to investigate whether such a computerized reporting system would improve the anesthesia provider's adherence to clinical guidelines. The first automated analysis showed that 70% of all surgical patients received antibiotics as per the accepted guideline. The AIMS database tracked antibiotic administration and generated reports from the database to provide specific feedback to individual care providers. Further analysis found that ORs that required extensive surgical setup, positioning, and anesthetic induction, such as cardiac surgery, neurosurgery, and orthopedic surgery, were less likely to be compliant with the antibiotics guideline. After 1 year of implementing the system, 92% of the eligible patients received antibiotics as per the accepted guideline.[16] However, further analysis was not done in this study to explain the residual nonadherence rate of 8% and determine the factors that prevented the ORs from reaching the desired compliance of greater than 99%. Nevertheless, the key element of success in this project was that the individual anesthesia providers were not merely being reported and forced to change their practice; instead, they were able to view and compare their own performance with other providers in a blinded method.[16]

By monitoring individual clinical practice patterns, AIMS can, in some circumstances, provide quality control and ensure compliance to standards and recommended guidelines. Even in cases when there are no adverse events, processes and behaviors can be improved.[15]

AIMS-BASED DECISION SUPPORT TO IMPROVE QUALITY
Reminders for Adherence to Clinical Guidelines

Physicians tend to be poorly compliant with published recommendations.[30–34] To assist with adherence, AIMS also have the ability to provide real-time decision support during the perioperative period in ways that can have a significant effect on quality. For example, AIMS-based alerts have been created to remind the clinicians shortly after the induction of anesthesia to provide prophylactic antibiotics, if none have been documented in the chart.[35] Likewise, an AIMS can improve prophylaxis for nausea and vomiting. Kooij and colleagues[36] found that at baseline, 38% of patients at high risk of postoperative nausea and vomiting were prescribed prophylaxis. After the introduction of an electronic decision support, the rate increased to 73% and decreased back to 37% when the system was removed.

At the Massachusetts General Hospital, the practice of maintaining intraoperative normothermia has been studied and modified using data collected by the AIMS. In each OR, the AIMS automatically records temperature information when a temperature probe is connected to the physiologic monitor.[3] When the temperature is less than a certain threshold (36°C), the providers then receive a prompt (**Fig. 2**) to encourage them to take additional action to maintain normothermia (such as by applying forced air warming devices or connecting an in-line fluid warmer).

Using the same automatic reminder capability, a potential area where AIMS can be useful perioperatively is in providing drug redosing reminders. For example, repeated anticoagulation is often required during prolonged vascular surgery. In other circumstances, patients may need redosing of multiple antibiotics with different administration schedules after the start of the surgery. In these scenarios, an accurate and dependable system that prompts the provider to complete certain clinical tasks may be effective in improving quality and reducing patient morbidity, particularly

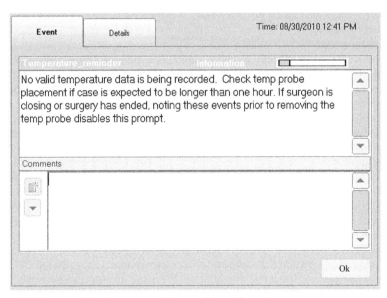

Fig. 2. AIMS-based notification on avoidance of hypothermia.

when clinicians are being asked to administer drugs that are only occasionally encountered in their practice (**Fig. 3**).

Operational Decision Support

To help clinicians achieve better adherence with clinical guidelines, AIMS can facilitate improvements in patient flow and operational throughout under the right circumstances. In addition, AIMS can improve institutional resource use by assisting in

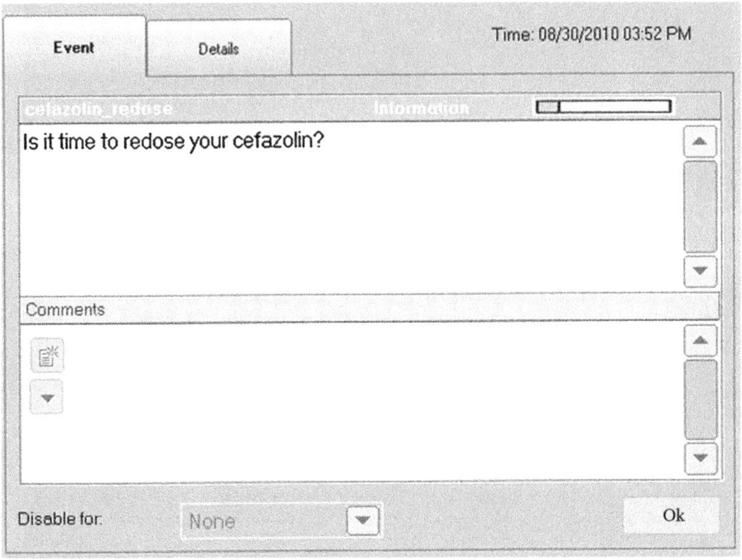

Fig. 3. AIMS-based drug redosing alert.

many different tracking functions that would be otherwise tedious and imprecise when performed manually.

One major area in which tracking is able to improve drug use is in the evaluation of pharmaceutical wastes. Gillerman and colleagues[37] recorded drug waste data for 6 anesthetic drugs commonly used in their department using an AIMS (atracurium, thiopental, succinylcholine, propofol, midazolam, and rocuronium) for 25,481 patients over 1 year and surveyed the providers' knowledge of departmental drug waste. The investigators discovered that the total cost of unadministered study drugs was $165,667, which was 26% of the expenditure for all drugs.[37] The reason most cited for drug waste was the disposal of full, or partially full, syringes.[37] More surprisingly, anesthesia providers in this study were found to have a correct perception of relative cost of drugs such as thiopental but thought that there was little need to conserve it. The data collected raised the issue that perhaps smaller multidose vials should be used than large stock solutions. In addition, education of providers about the use, waste, and cost of drugs was found to be helpful because these perceptions influenced handling of drug waste and conservation behaviors.

AIMS data have also been used by some investigators to assess how efficiently an OR is being run. For instance, the time when a patient enters and leaves the OR can be accurately tracked and used by OR managers to reallocate resources, identify ORs in which the turnover is problematic, or otherwise manage patient flow.[3,6]

At the Massachusetts General Hospital, AIMS is able to facilitate OR throughput via a custom display that has been installed in the anesthesia workroom (**Fig. 4**). This display allows anesthesia technicians to track the status of all 51 ORs. The technicians also receive automatic alert pages, generated by the AIMS, when cases are finishing. Other hospitals, notably the Thomas Jefferson University, the University of Michigan, and Vanderbilt University have used their AIMS to send automatic notifications regarding patient flow to the OR team. Notifications have ranged from "patient arrived in holding area" to "patient ready for surgery" and "next scheduled case cancelled."[3]

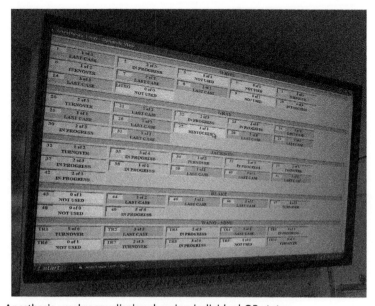

Fig. 4. Anesthesia workroom display showing individual OR status.

Detection of Outliers

Because the only means to compare the practice patterns of individual providers is often from the information in the anesthetic records, it is impractical to perform these kinds of analyses in the absence of an AIMS. Manual records maintained by different anesthesiologists are inconsistent, and the information recorded is often biased, as previously discussed. However, AIMS can provide automatically acquired objective data to assess the practice patterns of individual providers. These data can then be used by quality managers to detect outliers and drive performance improvement efforts.[12]

Improving the Quality of Information Transfer

Accurate and complete documentation is important for a variety of reasons, including ensuring the highest quality care,[16,18] transferring the information,[38,39] and facilitating provider reimbursement.[22] Although a patient may, in some circumstances, receive perfect medical care, if the corresponding documentation is flawed or insufficient, the efforts of the provider may not be recognized or financially reimbursed.[40] It is estimated that the average physician loses approximately 10% of potential revenue because of billing mistakes made at the point of care.[41] Furthermore, when one anesthesiologist hands over a case to another, the continuity of the care is critically important, and complete intraoperative records are essential for full information transfer.[42] Because AIMS can facilitate complete and accurate electronic charting, they have the capacity to improve information transfer and reduce the rate of missing information.[43]

Cost-Effectiveness

To date, there have been no studies on the overall cost-effectiveness of AIMS published in the peer-reviewed literature. Although it is difficult to calculate the overall benefit to patients in terms of more traditional measures (ie, lives saved per dollar spent), the benefits of these systems to patients have been proven in several areas.[3] AIMS have clearly been shown to enable clinicians to provide patients with appropriate care, mostly through their decision support tools, and may ultimately be shown to have cost-saving potential.

The Duke University Medical Center Department of Anesthesia used their AIMS to compute the costs of each anesthetic administered, and this information was used to reduce the average cost of an anesthetic from $56 to $32 per case. This cost reduction is estimated to have saved US $938,000 in the first year of its cost-containment program.[40]

LIMITATION OF AIMS

One of the potential and important downfalls of AIMS that affects quality control is the inability of the system to discern what data represent artifact in a particular clinical setting.[21] For example, the transducer for an arterial line may be momentarily dropped onto the ground and, thus, the AIMS would falsely record an abnormal value.[44] This false value may subsequently be interpreted as a clinically significant event. In another instance, a patient may experience transient desaturation from sedation but may quickly return to full saturation within a minute. With an electronic record, this event may be misinterpreted as a critical incident should there be a bad outcome, even if the event was unrelated to the momentary desaturation.[44,45] To address this problem, some AIMS require the user to validate physiologic values and other AIMS generate a confirmation button that allows the user to agree or disagree when a value is detected that is grossly outside of the normal ranges. For example, the Vanderbilt Perioperative Information Management System is one such system that requires users to validate vital signs before placing them into the electronic record.

Because the anesthesia record is a primary piece of evidence used in court during a malpractice proceeding, artifactual or transient data have significant medicolegal implications.[44] Feldman sent surveys to anesthesia departments in North America that used AIMS.[44] The survey was designed to investigate whether the use of AIMS increase malpractice exposure. Contrary to the concern that AIMS may increase liability, results showed that it is actually a useful risk-management tool. In fact, some investigators think that AIMS could be used to prevent litigations by helping to identify unsafe practices before the lawsuit occurs.[44]

One final criticism of AIMS, and all clinical decision support systems in general, is the degree to which providers become dependent on them. This dependence is problematic when systems fail or providers change institutions or clinical environments and no longer have access to the systems on which they have become reliant.[46]

FUTURE OF AIMS AND QUALITY PROCESS MEASURES

Although the utility and place of AIMS in the perioperative environment is wide ranging and fast growing, the current literature is still limited. Studies on AIMS have only been done in a few institutions because the widespread adoption of these technologies has not yet occurred worldwide. Trends from the past decade suggest that the penetration of AIMS will increase in the near future. AIMS have been demonstrated to be able to increase the quality of care and improve OR efficiency.[3,8,10,15,16] In addition, they have the capacity to alter the behavior of anesthesia providers and change clinical practice.[19] Enhancing the accuracy of intraoperative charting systems and easing information retrieval has the potential of enormous research and legal implications.

The most exciting and fastest area of AIMS product development is real-time clinical decision support. This feature has the potential to revolutionize the delivery of patient care by assisting clinicians in making the best clinical decision possible, while following the recommended practices. For example, one proposed system, on detection of a chaotic electrocardiogram and disappearance of a pulse oximeter waveform, could prompt the end user to consider ventricular fibrillation as a diagnostic possibility and then make the appropriate Advanced Cardiovascular Life Support algorithm available on-screen.[3] As these systems become more robust, eventually they will enable providers across a wide variety of scenarios to provide care in more effective and efficient ways.

REFERENCES

1. Bloomfield EL, Feinglass NG. The anesthesia information management system for electronic documentation: what are we waiting for? J Anesth 2008;22(4): 404–11.
2. Benson M, Junger A, Quinzio L, et al. Clinical and practical requirements of online software for anesthesia documentation an experience report. Int J Med Inform 2000;57(2/3):155–64.
3. Ehrenfeld JM, Rehman MA. Anesthesia information management systems: a review of functionality and installation considerations. J Clin Monit Comput 2010. [Epub ahead of print].

4. Egger Halbeis CB, Epstein RH, Macario A, et al. Adoption of anesthesia information management systems by academic departments in the United States. Anesth Analg 2008;107(4):1323–9.
5. Ehrenfeld JM. Anesthesia information management systems—a guide to their successful installation and use. Anesthesiology News September 2009;1–7.
6. Balust J, Egger Halbeis CB, Macario A. Prevalence of anaesthesia information management systems in university-affiliated hospitals in Europe. Eur J Anaesthesiol 2010;27(2):202–8.
7. Boersma E, Kertai MD, Schouten O, et al. Perioperative cardiovascular mortality in noncardiac surgery: validation of the Lee Cardiac Risk Index. Am J Med 2005; 118(10):1134–41.
8. Edsall DW, Deshane P, Giles C, et al. Computerized patient anesthesia records: less time and better quality than manually produced anesthesia records. J Clin Anesth 1993;5(4):275–83.
9. Rohrig R, Junger A, Hartmann B, et al. The incidence and prediction of automatically detected intraoperative cardiovascular events in noncardiac surgery. Anesth Analg 2004;98(3):569–77.
10. Bates DW, Gawande AA. Improving safety with information technology. N Engl J Med 2003;348(25):2526–34.
11. Sandberg WS, Sandberg EH, Seim AR, et al. Real-time checking of electronic anesthesia records for documentation errors and automatically text messaging clinicians improves quality of documentation. Anesth Analg 2008;106(1): 192–201.
12. Muravchick S, Caldwell JE, Epstein RH, et al. Anesthesia information management system implementation: a practical guide. Anesth Analg 2008;107(5): 1598–608.
13. Benson M, Junger A, Fuchs C, et al. Using an anesthesia information management system to prove a deficit in voluntary reporting of adverse events in a quality assurance program. J Clin Monit Comput 2000;16(3):211–7.
14. Lerou JG, Dirksen R, van Daele M, et al. Automated charting of physiological variables in anesthesia: a quantitative comparison of automated versus handwritten anesthesia records. J Clin Monit 1988;4(1):37–47.
15. Balust J, Macario A. Can anesthesia information management systems improve quality in the surgical suite? Curr Opin Anaesthesiol 2009;22(2):215–22.
16. O'Reilly M, Talsma A, VanRiper S, et al. An anesthesia information system designed to provide physician-specific feedback improves timely administration of prophylactic antibiotics. Anesth Analg 2006;103(4):908–12.
17. Driscoll WD, Columbia MA, Peterfreund RA. An observational study of anesthesia record completeness using an anesthesia information management system. Anesth Analg 2007;104(6):1454–61.
18. Hollenberg JP, Pirraglia PA, Williams-Russo P, et al. Computerized data collection in the operating room during coronary artery bypass surgery: a comparison to the hand-written anesthesia record. J Cardiothorac Vasc Anesth 1997;11(5):545–51.
19. Ehrenfeld JM, Sandberg WS. Incidence of intraoperative gaps in patient monitoring during anesthesia. Anesthesiology 2006;A974.
20. Benson M, Junger A, Quinzio L, et al. Influence of the method of data collection on the documentation of blood-pressure readings with an Anesthesia Information Management System (AIMS). Methods Inf Med 2001;40(3):190–5.
21. Cook RI, McDonald JS, Nunziata E. Differences between handwritten and automatic blood pressure records. Anesthesiology 1989;71(3):385–90.

22. Reich DL, Wood RK Jr, Mattar R, et al. Arterial blood pressure and heart rate discrepancies between handwritten and computerized anesthesia records. Anesth Analg 2000;91(3):612–6.
23. Ouchterlony J, Arvidsson S, Sjostedt L, et al. Peroperative and immediate postoperative adverse events in patients undergoing elective general and orthopaedic surgery. The Gothenburg study of perioperative risk (PROPER). Part II. Acta Anaesthesiol Scand 1995;39(5):643–52.
24. Cohen MM, Duncan PG, Pope WD, et al. The Canadian four-centre study of anaesthetic outcomes: II. Can outcomes be used to assess the quality of anaesthesia care? Can J Anaesth 1992;39(5 Pt 1):430–9.
25. Cohen MM, Duncan PG, Pope WD, et al. A survey of 112,000 anaesthetics at one teaching hospital (1975–83). Can Anaesth Soc J 1986;33(1):22–31.
26. Cooper JB, Cullen DJ, Nemeskal R, et al. Effects of information feedback and pulse oximetry on the incidence of anesthesia complications. Anesthesiology 1987;67(5):686–94.
27. Forrest JB, Rehder K, Cahalan MK, et al. Multicenter study of general anesthesia. III. Predictors of severe perioperative adverse outcomes. Anesthesiology 1992;76(1): 3–15.
28. Beilin Y, Wax D, Torrillo T, et al. A survey of anesthesiologists' and nurses' attitudes toward the implementation of an Anesthesia Information Management System on a labor and delivery floor. Int J Obstet Anesth 2009;18(1):22–7.
29. Vigoda MM, Gencorelli F, Lubarsky DA. Changing medical group behaviors: increasing the rate of documentation of quality assurance events using an anesthesia information system. Anesth Analg 2006;103(2):390–5.
30. Sanborn KV, Castro J, Kuroda M, et al. Detection of intraoperative incidents by electronic scanning of computerized anesthesia records. Comparison with voluntary reporting. Anesthesiology 1996;85(5):977–87.
31. Costanza ME, Stoddard AM, Zapka JG, et al. Physician compliance with mammography guidelines: barriers and enhancers. J Am Board Fam Pract 1992;5(2):143–52.
32. Headrick LA, Speroff T, Pelecanos HI, et al. Efforts to improve compliance with the National Cholesterol Education Program guidelines. Results of a randomized controlled trial. Arch Intern Med 1992;152(12):2490–6.
33. Browner WS, Baron RB, Solkowitz S, et al. Physician management of hypercholesterolemia. A randomized trial of continuing medical education. West J Med 1994;161(6):572–8.
34. Studnicki J, Schapira DV, Bradham DD, et al. Response to the National Cancer Institute Alert. The effect of practice guidelines on two hospitals in the same medical community. Cancer 1993;72(10):2986–92.
35. Cohen MM, Rose DK, Yee DA. Changing anesthesiologists' practice patterns. Can it be done? Anesthesiology 1996;85(2):260–9.
36. Kooij FO, Klok T, Hollmann MW, et al. Decision support increases guideline adherence for prescribing postoperative nausea and vomiting prophylaxis. Anesth Analg 2008;106(3):893–8.
37. Gillerman RG, Browning RA. Drug use inefficiency: a hidden source of wasted health care dollars. Anesth Analg 2000;91(4):921–4.
38. Fuchs C, Quinzio L, Benson M, et al. Integration of a handheld based anaesthesia rounding system into an anaesthesia information management system. Int J Med Inform 2006;75(7):553–63.
39. Epstein RH, Ekbatani A, Kaplan J, et al. Development of a staff recall system for mass casualty incidents using cell phone text messaging. Anesth Analg 2010; 110(3):871–8.

40. Girbes AR, Zijlstra JG. Spend time on patients and families or on documentation? Anesth Analg 2009;109(3):691–2.
41. Terry K. How the device in your hand can put more money in your pocket. Med Econ 2001;78(24):44–6, 49–50.
42. O'Byrne WT 3rd, Weavind L, Selby J. The science and economics of improving clinical communication. Anesthesiol Clin 2008;26(4):729–44, vii.
43. Meyer-Bender A, Spitz R, Pollwein B. The anaesthetic report: custom-made print-outs from anaesthesia-information-management-systems using extensible style-sheet language transformation. J Clin Monit Comput 2010;24(1):51–60.
44. Feldman JM. Do anesthesia information systems increase malpractice exposure? Results of a survey. Anesth Analg 2004;99(3):840–3.
45. Ehrenfeld JM, Funk LM, Van Schalkwyk J, et al. The incidence of hypoxemia during surgery: evidence from two institutions. Can J Anaesth 2010;57(10): 888–97.
46. Chambers CV, Balaban DJ, Carlson BL, et al. The effect of microcomputer-generated reminders on influenza vaccination rates in a university based family practice center. J Am Board Fam Pract 1991;4:19–26.

Outcomes Research Using Quality Improvement Databases: Evolving Opportunities and Challenges

Satya Krishna Ramachandran, MD, FRCA*,
Sachin Kheterpal, MD, MBA

KEYWORDS

• Database • Quality improvement • Registry • Perioperative

THE EVOLUTION OF PERIOPERATIVE OUTCOMES RESEARCH

Anesthesia-related mortality has diminished over the last half century from about 1 in 1000 anesthesia procedures in the 1940s to 1 in 10000 in the 1970s and to 1 in 100,000 in the 1990s and early 2000s.[1] This reduction in catastrophic intraoperative events has largely been achieved through advances in technology, particularly pulse oximetry monitoring and end-tidal capnography. Although the traditional approach is to label complications occurring beyond the immediate postoperative period as surgical complications, a growing body of literature in small case series or animal models has demonstrated that the anesthetic management of intraoperative injury, stress, and inflammation may modify broad-ranging postoperative outcomes such as myocardial infarction, acute kidney injury, infection, venous thromboembolism, cancer progression, and cognitive decline.[2] So, as with perioperative beta-blockade[3] or with the evidence against aprotinin,[4] tools to broaden the focus from the prevention of rare events to the modulation of long-term outcomes have been developed in anesthesiology.

CHALLENGES IN EVALUATING THE EFFECTIVENESS OF INTRAOPERATIVE INTERVENTIONS

The need for research into the effect of anesthetic management stands in stark contrast to the many challenges that confront perioperative clinical research. The

Department of Anesthesiology, University of Michigan Medical School, 1 H427 University Hospital Box 0048, 1500 East Medical Center Drive, Ann Arbor, MI 48109-0048, USA
* Corresponding author.
E-mail address: rsatyak@med.umich.edu

Anesthesiology Clin 29 (2011) 71–81
doi:10.1016/j.anclin.2010.11.005
1932-2275/11/$ – see front matter © 2011 Elsevier Inc. All rights reserved.

perioperative period is a physically intrusive and expensive care setting. Patient and provider blinding during randomized trials is often impossible because of the invasive nature of the operation and anesthetic itself. The high throughput and focus on operational efficiency causes each minute of operative time to be measured, analyzed, and eliminated, often at the expense of important health care goals such as quality improvement (QI) and research. In addition, the ethical recruitment of patients is challenging in perioperative medicine, given the acuity of adverse events. For example, an institutional review board (IRB) is unlikely to approve randomization of patients to the control arm of an intraoperative blood pressure management study. However, a study of 15000 patients revealed that more than 40% of the patients experience profound hypotension in the operating room, defined as systolic blood pressure of 79 mm Hg or less.[5] Finally, the intraoperative period offers an overwhelming amount of information, dozens of vital signs and physiologic parameters every 60 seconds, that challenges classic manual data collection and analysis techniques. In aggregate, these challenges make traditional research techniques, such as the blinded randomized controlled trial, difficult to implement in the perioperative setting.

As a result, the perioperative specialties often require large multicenter randomized controlled trials to guide clinical decision making. Paradoxically, the effectiveness or complications associated with operative fundamentals such as surgical technique, open versus minimally invasive, and anesthesia type, sedation versus neuraxial versus general, are typically never even compared before widespread adoption. The 3 perioperative management strategies that were aggressively adopted because of landmark efficacy trials and are now questioned because of the increased risk of adverse events include use of aprotinin during cardiopulmonary bypass,[4] perioperative beta-blockade during noncardiac surgery,[3] and tight glucose level control in the postoperative period.[6] Each of these interventions demonstrated that large outcomes studies are necessary in perioperative patients to provide real-world risk and benefit information. Aprotinin was withdrawn from the market, the preoperative initiation of beta-blockade before noncardiac surgery remains controversial, and intensive care units now strive for serum glucose levels less than 180 mg/dL because of the conflicting effectiveness data published decades after the initial efficacy trials.

Even the current national clinical perioperative standards, such as the maintenance of normothermia to reduce surgical site infections, are based on small studies of a few hundred patients undergoing specific high-risk surgical procedures. These data are then extrapolated to broader patient populations and surgical procedures without interventional or observational data to support their adoption or guide their implementation.

THE NEED FOR QI DATA IN PERIOPERATIVE CLINICAL RESEARCH

The challenges to prospective randomized controlled trials has necessitated a the exploration of observational data sets that are capable of supporting robust research into the predictors and modulators of preoperative adverse events. The primary purpose and design of QI databases is quality assessment and improvement at the local, regional, or national level. However, these data can also provide the opportunity to robustly study specific questions related to patient outcomes with no additional clinical risk to the patient.

Conceptually, for a given operative procedure, variations in patient outcomes can be considered a result of the interaction among baseline preoperative patient risk, structure of care, and processes of care (**Fig. 1**). QI databases can be used to address the contribution of each of these 3 factors to variability in outcomes. However, the

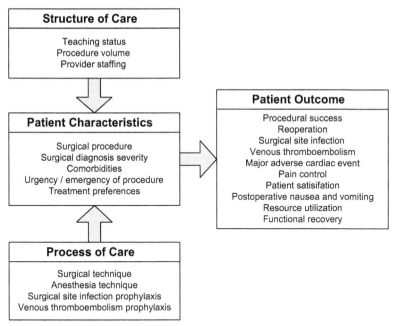

Fig. 1. Algorithm of variations in patient outcomes.

ability of a specific QI database to answer research questions regarding each of these factors is limited by the data elements collected in the QI effort. For example, investigations on the effect of process-of-care measures require data collection of detailed clinical intervention, such as medication administration, timing, and dosing. On the other hand, risk profiling and outcome prediction require patient comorbidities, operative risk, and outcome data.

A major goal of outcomes research rests in its desire to assess the relative benefit and risk associated with therapies. Large outcomes research efforts are statistically powered to detect not only the beneficial effects of an intervention but also the infrequent adverse events. This feature is qualitatively distinct from that of randomized controlled trials that primarily serve to detect the beneficial effect because the number of patients required for this end point is significantly smaller than that required for determining adverse effect causation. In addition, randomized controlled trials do not typically represent routine clinical practice. The inherent variability in routine provider care and patient factors allows for comparisons based on parameters that could be considered unethical in prospective randomized research methodology.

OVERVIEW OF THE EXISTING QI DATABASES

There are several QI databases that have been used by contemporary anesthesiology research. The strengths and weaknesses of these databases have been summarized in **Table 1**.

The Society of Thoracic Surgeons

In the late 1980s the Society of Thoracic Surgeons (STS) initially developed the STS National Adult Cardiac Surgery Database (STS NCD).[7] One of the first national surgical QI efforts, the STS collects detailed preoperative patient comorbidities, intraoperative

Table 1
Strengths and weaknesses of QI database research

Strengths	Weaknesses
Controlled and audited data collection improves data robustness	Focused sampling process limits understanding of other related conditions
Representative segment of patient population	Because of sampling methods, not a true measure of the breadth of care processes
Data elements are discreet, defined, and have validity	Not all data of value are collected in each database
Data element definitions are clear and aid both data collection and interpretation	Controlled definitions that do not evolve over time
Predefined outcomes variables	Outcomes cannot be modified to address a specific new research focus
Follow-up period stipulated, ensuring a standardized time-dependent outcome	Cannot obtain additional follow-up outcome data
Multicenter, representative of a broad cross-section	—
Limited IRB restraints	Resource intensive
Manual collection process limits data collection errors	Manual collection process is time consuming, expensive, and labor intensive

procedural interventions, and long-term postoperative outcomes. At the end of 2008, 892 sites participated and submitted data on 270,000 procedures annually. Rather than a random sampling methodology, all patients undergoing cardiac procedures are prospectively enrolled in the QI data collection process at each participating site. STS risk models have been developed for death and major morbidities including reoperation for any reason, permanent stroke, renal failure, deep sternal wound infection, prolonged ventilation time, and postoperative length of stay. These models are updated approximately every 3 years and are calibrated annually to make the expected (predicted) occurrences of each outcome equal to the national observed events for that year.[8] The STS NCD is widely considered one of the most mature and robust surgical QI efforts. Recently, STS risk-adjusted outcome comparisons were made available for lay public use, a first for national surgical QI databases.

The American College of Surgeons National Surgical Quality Improvement Program

The American College of Surgeons National Surgical Quality Improvement Program (ACS NSQIP) is a robust reporting system designed to provide reliable risk-adjusted surgical outcomes in a broadly representative national sample of general and vascular surgery patients.[9] More than 200 community hospitals, moderate-sized private hospitals, and tertiary care academic centers participated in the ACS NSQIP data collection and process improvement.[10] For each operation, a trained surgical clinical reviewer (typically a nurse) prospectively collects patient demographics, preoperative comorbidities, operative procedure information, limited intraoperative elements, and postoperative adverse occurrences up to 30 days after the operation. Surgical clinical reviewers undergo rigorous training and standardized testing before participation in data collection. They are trained on definitions and criteria for all 137 data elements collected for each ACS NSQIP case. In addition, a biennial data audit of each contributing center's data is performed by central ACS NSQIP staff. For the year 2008, a national audit demonstrated a low 1.36% discordance rate for more than 100,000 patient data elements reviewed.[11]

National Anesthesia Clinical Outcomes Registry

The National Anesthesia Clinical Outcomes Registry is a data warehouse that will eventually capture the 25 million anesthetics (a rough estimate) and millions of pain clinic procedures performed each year by anesthesiologists in the United States.[12] Data captured will eventually be divided into 4 categories:

1. Practice demographics, describing the anesthesia group (age, training, certifications, subspecialties) and the environment (hospital size, inpatient/outpatient mix).
2. Case-specific data in several tiers including simple (eg, current procedural terminology code, anesthesia type, provider code, patient age), moderate (eg, duration of surgery, agents used), and complex (eg, output from Anesthesia Information Management System with vital signs, fluids, drug doses).
3. Outcome data including basic (eg, intraoperative cancellation, mortality, major morbidities) and extended (eg, infections, prolonged length of stay, late events). The basis for recognized outcomes of interest will be the American Society of Anesthesiologists Committee on Performance and Outcomes Measurement definitions. Information will come from anesthesiology department data or from linkage to surgical databases that contain long-term patient outcome.
4. Risk adjustment data such as *International Classification of Diseases, Ninth Revision* diagnostic codes, preoperative medication use, defined comorbidities, hospital length of stay. Much of these data will come from the hospital or health care facility's systems.

The Society for Ambulatory Anesthesia Clinical Outcomes Registry

The Society for Ambulatory Anesthesia Clinical Outcomes Registry is a database directed at collecting case-specific data using online and mobile data entry forms. The database is in evolution and is expected to provide national comparative data, which may be of significant QI value to local contributing hospitals.

National Registry of Cardiopulmonary Resuscitation

The National Registry of Cardiopulmonary Resuscitation (NRCPR) is a prospective, observational, multicenter registry of in-hospital cardiac arrests.[13] Hospitals join voluntarily and pay a fee for data support and quarterly QI reports. Hospital medical records of sequential cardiac arrests are abstracted electronically by trained NRCPR-certified research coordinators at each institution. Data elements use standardized Utstein nomenclature to facilitate consistent definitions of variables across multiple sites. Data abstractors are required to successfully complete a certification examination. These examinations comprise evaluation of data abstraction, entry accuracy, and operational definition compliance before a site is allowed to submit data to the NRCPR. In addition, the data entry software (provided by Digital Innovation Inc, Forest Hill, Maryland, USA, 2008) has more than 300 checks and smart skips to assist with accurate data entry. Participating hospitals are required to submit 10% of their resuscitation forms so that reabstraction can be performed by NRCPR personnel. Other efforts to ensure data accuracy include ongoing abstractor training with monthly user's group calls and an annual user's group conference. Six major categories of variables for each patient with a cardiac arrest are collected, including (1) facility data, (2) patient demographic data, (3) preevent data, (4) event data, (5) outcome data, and (6) process QI data.

THE VALUE OF SURGICAL QI DATA IN PERIOPERATIVE RESEARCH

Given the paucity of randomized controlled trial data in perioperative research, QI data play a prominent role in advancement of this field. QI data offer insight into 3 important areas including risk prediction and patient consent, assessment of practice and outcome variation, and enabling future research efforts. Fundamentally, the informed consent process for health care delivery involves communicating the reasonable risks and benefits involved with a health care intervention. QI data enable research that allows for data-informed consent processes. Rather than generic comments regarding the range of possible outcomes, basic QI research allows us to identify patients at low or high risk for perioperative morbidity and mortality. Although a given patient's outcome cannot be predicted using QI research, the patient's preoperative comorbidities and planned operative procedure can be compared with national or local data to provide the patient and surgeon relative risk information. For example, among patients undergoing general surgery, the risk of acute kidney injury is increased 3-fold by the presence of preoperative ascites and 2-fold by the observation of active congestive heart failure.[14] This information was obtained using QI data and provided the first data regarding the effect of specific preoperative conditions on the risk of acute kidney injury after general surgery, an understudied area of research.

Next, although much of medical research is based on identifying interventions with high efficacy, it remains clear that the real-world implementation of these interventions often lags behind the evidence demonstrating their value. There continues to be wide variations in care patterns and outcomes for the same interventional procedure. Researchers may hypothesize regarding the underlying cause of variation, but the ability to identify the variation itself is an important contribution of QI data research. For example, national bodies have published specific recommendations for the use of thrombolytic therapy versus percutaneous coronary intervention for acute myocardial infarction. However, a recent analysis of national registry data demonstrates that many patients who would have benefited from percutaneous coronary intervention did not receive it.[15] More importantly, neither patient nor clinical factors explain the wide range in the use of optimal therapy. These QI data demonstrate the important need for further research into the gap between optimal and actual care.

Finally, QI data research enables future interventional research by providing researchers with the necessary preliminary work to target specific high-risk patient populations, procedures, or processes. QI data allow researchers to perform a data biopsy of the current practice patterns and outcomes. Given the challenges of conducting prospective randomized controlled trials in perioperative medicine, exploratory analyses using QI data are an essential component of the scientific method. For example, initial hypotheses regarding an adverse relationship between the age of red blood cells and outcomes in cardiac surgery were first assessed using observational single-center QI data.[16] These data demonstrated a compelling relationship that is now being evaluated using a prospective randomized controlled trial (Red Cell Storage Duration and Outcomes in Cardiac Surgery, ClinicalTrials.gov identifier: NCT0045878). However, without the initial QI data research, it is unlikely that the interventional trial would have been funded, passed IRB review, or provided a compelling controversy for patient enrollment.

LIMITATIONS OF EXISTING QI DATA

National surgical outcome registries, such as the ACS NSQIP and STS databases, have demonstrated their ability as QI, benchmarking, risk prediction, and hypothesis-generating tools. Their highly reliable preoperative risk stratification and 30-day postoperative outcomes data have been used to evaluate the relationship between hospital structure, comorbidities, and patient outcomes. However, these databases have struggled to provide data usable for outcomes research for several reasons. First, although manual data collection by a trained clinician creates highly reliable data, prospective registries are forced to take a parsimonious approach to database element selection because of the high cost of the manual process itself.[17] For example, although the ACS NSQIP collects 137 data elements for every case, essential clinical interventions such as preoperative medications, intraoperative medications and physiologic data, and postoperative interventions are completely absent. As a result, although the data from these registries inform analyses of structures of care, they cannot provide data on the comparative effectiveness of specific clinical interventions.

In addition, these registries struggle to evolve as the clinical questions and state of knowledge advance. Detailed definitions for each clinical element must be tested and evaluated across a broad range of users, patients, and cases. Any change requires manual training across hundreds of data collectors and sites. Therefore, contemporary clinical questions are often unanswerable because of outdated definitions or absent clinical elements. For example, despite the current importance of health care–associated infections, the ACS NSQIP lacks any data regarding perioperative prophylactic antibiotics, maintenance of normothermia, or proper hair removal. In addition, the ACS NSQIP does not incorporate serum cardiac injury biomarkers into its definition of perioperative cardiac adverse events despite national standards advocating the use of biomarkers. Finally, expansion of existing registry efforts is cost prohibitive. Annual ACS NSQIP participation and data collection costs are at least $120,000 and only allow for collection of data on approximately 1500 patients per hospital per year.[18] Payer underwriting in the hopes of improved outcomes have resulted in increased participation in some states. Expanding the manual data collection to the remaining cases at a given facility or increasing the number of elements tracked could cost millions of dollars per year. In addition, a manual registry process does not scale over time, given that participation and data collection costs do not decrease over time. The Acute Physiology and Chronic Health Evaluation (APACHE) critical care experience demonstrates that expensive manual registries may fade after an initial adoption phase. In order to collect data comprehensively, automated data collection processes are essential.

LEGAL AND ETHICAL CHALLENGES

Registry data are traditionally used for QI activities but have increasing research use, with several high-impact journal publications in the recent years. This use creates unique challenges with regard to patient confidentiality and regulatory requirements. The Belmont Report in 1979[19] identified 3 fundamental ethical principles for human subject research. These principles are respect for persons, beneficence, and justice. Together these principles provide a foundation for the ethical analysis of human subjects research, including the use of health information in registries developed for scientific purposes with a prospect of producing social benefits. The following are the federal regulations that apply to research on registries:

1. The Privacy Rule (derived from 45 CFR §160 and §164), which specifically addresses security and privacy considerations regarding individually identifiable patient information, referred to as Protected Health Information (PHI) by the Privacy Rule. The Privacy Rule requirements apply to any research that requires PHI, whether it is federally related or not.

2. The Common Rule, derived from subpart A of 45 CFR §46. This Common Rule is used as an overarching regulatory principle governing human subjects research conducted, supported, or otherwise subject to regulation by any federal department or agency "45 CFR §46.101(a)," and it includes requirements for IRB review and patient informed consent. Although the Common Rule only regulates federally supported research, many academic medical centers apply the Common Rule to all research by policy.

IS AN IRB REVIEW REQUIRED

Although use of QI data is widespread, there are many misconceptions regarding the IRB's scope of oversight for QI data.[20] Because QI is considered a core function of a health care enterprise, patient consent and IRB approval is not required for QI initiatives themselves. However, if QI data are used for publication in the peer-reviewed literature, an IRB review of the project is essential. Although the project may eventually be deemed exempt and not require subsequent annual IRB consideration, this assessment must be made by the IRB, not the principal investigator. The 3 basic questions that are to be used to ascertain the need for an IRB review and informed consent are

1. Are the data intended to be used for research? Even if research was not the original primary purpose, the use of data for research or publication automatically necessitates a formal IRB review.
2. Are human subjects or their data involved? Human subjects research refers to data collected through intervention or interaction with the individual or identifiable private information. This form of research requires an IRB review to adjudicate on the need for informed consent and Health Insurance Portability and Accountability Act (HIPAA) authorization.
3. Is informed consent required? Waiver of informed consent is possible if the following criteria are satisfied:
   • The research involves no more than minimal risk to the subjects.
   • The waiver or alteration will not adversely affect the rights and welfare of the subjects.
   • The research could not practicably be performed without the waiver or alteration.
   • Whenever appropriate, the subjects will be provided with additional pertinent information after participation.

CONSIDERATIONS FOR STUDY DESIGN USING QI DATA

Randomized controlled trials require rigorous study design before initiating the trial. Similarly, observational research using QI data also demands specific efforts to maximize scientific validity and integrity (**Table 2**).[21]

Defining the Study Population

In order to establish a robust study, one of the essential steps is to first define appropriate inclusion and exclusion criteria. The inclusion criteria generally include geographic, demographic, disease-specific, or temporal criteria that broadly capture the breadth and scope of the study population of interest. Exclusion criteria, on the other hand, are used to concentrate the study efforts on a tightly defined section of the population. An equally important step is accurately defining the study groups. One method is to use process-of-care measures that are readily understandable and clinically applicable. An example is the use of timing of defibrillation as the

Table 2	
Considerations for study design	
Construct	**Relevant Questions**
Research question	What are the clinical questions of interest
Study design	What types of study designs can be used in registries
Exposures and outcomes	How do the clinical questions of interest translate into measurable exposures and outcomes
Study population	What types of patients are needed for study Is a comparison group needed How should patients be selected for study
Data sources	Where can the necessary data be found
Study size and duration	For how long should data be collected and for how many patients
Potential for bias	What is the potential for bias, and how does this affect generalizability (external validity)

From Gliklich RE, Dreyer NA, editors. Registries for evaluating patient outcomes: a user's guide. (Prepared by Outcome DEcIDE Center [Outcome Sciences, Incorporated dba Outcome] under Contract No. HHSA290200500035I TO1.) AHRQ Publication No. 07-EHC001-1. Rockville (MD): Agency for Healthcare Research and Quality; April 2007.

process-of-care measure to establish the effect of delayed treatment on survival to hospital discharge.[22] In this study, the comparative groups were determined by the presence or absence of delayed defibrillation. A more commonly used method is to define comparative groups based on the presence or absence of disease process.[23,24]

Several methods have been described in the literature to ensure adequate sample size for observational analyses, such as those using QI data. If a logistic regression model is required to assess the relationship between independent variables and a dichotomous dependent outcome of interest, the critical factors are the number of outcome events and the number of independent variables of interest. It is generally accepted that overfitting-adjusted risk models with more than one variable per 10 outcome events will result in the generation of spurious associations. So, for example, a collection of 140 events will permit the inclusion of up to 14 variables into a logistic regression model without the risk of overfitting. Conversely, if there are 18 variables of interest and only 140 events, the study does not have adequate sample size to ensure robust prediction modeling.

Defining the Study End Points

An important step in using QI databases involves choosing outcome measures that are of clinical value and dependable either because of nature of data (laboratory values) or because of robust data handling processes (NSQIP outcomes). Thus, QI research end points such as acute renal failure defined by absolute creatinine values,[24] cardiac adverse events defined by serum biomarker values,[25] and survival to discharge after cardiopulmonary resuscitation[22] have been used successfully in the literature. In determining the robustness of end points, it is essential to establish that the follow-up was obtained equally across comparison groups. In other words, creatinine values may be used to determine acute renal failure, but absence of a value does not mean absence of renal failure. As a result, inclusion of variables with significant missing data in the analysis carries a significant risk of spurious study conclusions.

Handling Missing Data

Missing data affects study validity by both reducing the information yield of the study and, in many cases, introducing bias. Missing data are classified depending on whether missing is a random occurrence.[26] Random missing data influence study strength but generally do not introduce bias. It may be necessary to demonstrate the absence of bias by using adjusted modeling techniques. If there are significant differences in the distribution of observed variables for patients with specific missing data to the distribution of those variables for patients for whom those same data are present, it can generally be surmised that the missing data will influence the validity of the study findings. Thus it is essential to report the proportion of complete data for each variable of interest.[21]

Ensuring Data Integrity

Interrater variability in interpretation or coding of specific conditions results in erroneous data. Errors in data entry occur when data are entered into the registry inaccurately, for example, a laboratory value of 2.0 is entered as 20.[21] Errors of intention refer to the intentional distortion of data to improve on-site performance of risk-adjusted outcomes or selecting only cases with good outcomes. Before using the data from any QI database, one should ensure that there are adequate quality checks of the data that include, at the very least, testing and reporting on interrater reliability and reabstraction.

In conclusion, although outcomes-based registries and databases can provide useful information, there are levels of rigor that enhance validity and make the information from some registries more useful for guiding decisions than the information from others. The virtual explosion of anesthesia-related registries has opened seemingly limitless opportunities for outcomes research. These research opportunities include areas traditionally considered unsuitable for prospective randomized trials in addition to generating hypothesis for more rigorous prospective analysis.

REFERENCES

1. Li G, Warner M, Lang BH, et al. Epidemiology of anesthesia-related mortality in the United States, 1999–2005. Anesthesiology 2009;110:759–65.
2. Sessler DI. Long-term consequences of anesthetic management. Anesthesiology 2009;111:1–4.
3. Devereaux PJ, Yang H, Yusuf S, et al. Effects of extended-release metoprolol succinate in patients undergoing non-cardiac surgery (POISE trial): a randomised controlled trial. Lancet 2008;371:1839–47.
4. Ray WA. Learning from aprotinin–mandatory trials of comparative efficacy and safety needed. N Engl J Med 2008;358:840–2.
5. Bijker JB, van Klei WA, Kappen TH, et al. Incidence of intraoperative hypotension as a function of the chosen definition: literature definitions applied to a retrospective cohort using automated data collection. Anesthesiology 2007;107:213–20.
6. Finfer S, Chittock DR, Su SY, et al. Intensive versus conventional glucose control in critically ill patients. N Engl J Med 2009;360:1283–97.
7. Edwards FH. The STS database at 20 years: a tribute to Dr Richard E. Clark. Ann Thorac Surg 2010;89:9–10.
8. Jin R, Furnary AP, Fine SC, et al. Using Society of Thoracic Surgeons risk models for risk-adjusting cardiac surgery results. Ann Thorac Surg 2010;89:677–82.
9. Khuri SF, Daley J, Henderson W, et al. The Department of Veterans Affairs' NSQIP: the first national, validated, outcome-based, risk-adjusted, and peer-controlled

program for the measurement and enhancement of the quality of surgical care. National VA Surgical Quality Improvement Program. Ann Surg 1998;228:491–507.

10. Khuri SF, Henderson WG, Daley J, et al. Successful implementation of the Department of Veterans Affairs' National Surgical Quality Improvement Program in the private sector: the Patient Safety in Surgery study. Ann Surg 2008;248:329–36.

11. Shiloach M, Frencher SK Jr, Steeger JE, et al. Toward robust information: data quality and inter-rater reliability in the American College of Surgeons National Surgical Quality Improvement Program. J Am Coll Surg 2010;210:6–16.

12. Available at: http://www.aqihq.org/NACORIntro.aspx. Accessed October 8, 2010.

13. Peberdy MA, Kaye W, Ornato JP, et al. Cardiopulmonary resuscitation of adults in the hospital: a report of 14720 cardiac arrests from the National Registry of Cardiopulmonary Resuscitation. Resuscitation 2003;58:297–308.

14. Kheterpal S, Tremper KK, Heung M, et al. Development and validation of an acute kidney injury risk index for patients undergoing general surgery: results from a national data set. Anesthesiology 2009;110:505–15.

15. Khawaja FJ, Ting HH. Quality dimensions of primary percutaneous coronary intervention: timeliness, access, and availability. Circulation 2009;120:2411–3.

16. Koch CG, Li L, Sessler DI, et al. Duration of red-cell storage and complications after cardiac surgery. N Engl J Med 2008;358:1229–39.

17. Nathan H, Pawlik TM. Limitations of claims and registry data in surgical oncology research. Ann Surg Oncol 2008;15:415–23.

18. American College of Surgeons National Surgical Quality Improvement Program (ACS NSQIP): Seminannual Report. Chicago (IL), July 1, 2007 through June 30, 2008, 2009.

19. National Commission for the Potection of Human Subjects of Biomedical and Behavioral Research. The Belmont Report: ethical principles and guidelines for the protection of human subjects of research. Washington, DC: US Government Printing Office; 1979.

20. Dokholyan RS, Muhlbaier LH, Falletta JM, et al. Regulatory and ethical considerations for linking clinical and administrative databases. Am Heart J 2009;157: 971–82.

21. Gliklich RE, Dreyer NA, editors. Registries for evaluating patient outcomes: a user's guide. (Prepared by Outcome DEcIDE Center [Outcome Sciences, Inc dba Outcome] under Contract No. HHSA290200500035I TO1.) AHRQ Publication No. 07-EHC001-1. Rockville (MD): Agency for Healthcare Research and Quality; 2007.

22. Mhyre JM, Ramachandran SK, Kheterpal S, et al. Delayed time to defibrillation after intraoperative and periprocedural cardiac arrest. Anesthesiology 2010; 113:782–93.

23. Ramachandran SK, Kheterpal S, Consens F, et al. Derivation and validation of a simple perioperative sleep apnea prediction score. Anesth Analg 2010;110: 1007–15.

24. Kheterpal S, Tremper KK, Englesbe MJ, et al. Predictors of postoperative acute renal failure after noncardiac surgery in patients with previously normal renal function. Anesthesiology 2007;107:892–902.

25. Kheterpal S, O'Reilly M, Englesbe MJ, et al. Preoperative and intraoperative predictors of cardiac adverse events after general, vascular, and urological surgery. Anesthesiology 2009;110:58–66.

26. Little R, Rubin D. Statistical analysis with missing data. New York: John Wiley & Sons; 1987.

Preventing Postoperative Complications in the Elderly

Frederick E. Sieber, MD[a,b,*], Sheila Ryan Barnett, MD[c,d]

KEYWORDS

- Geriatric • Surgery • Delirium
- Surgical procedures/Adverse effects
- Postoperative complications • Quality assurance • Aged

The population is aging because better medical care and living conditions have allowed people to reach an older age in better health than previously possible.[1] As the elderly have continued to increase in number, so has the number of surgical procedures performed on this segment of the population. Orthopedic surgery provides an example of this phenomenon. From 1990 to 2004, the number of total hip arthroplasties performed increased by 158%.[2] Adjusted rates of cervical spine fusions in the elderly increased by 206% from 1992 to 2005.[3] In the Medicare population, from 1979 to 1992, rates of surgery for spinal stenosis increased 8-fold.[4] Other surgical specialties, such as urology, have seen similar changes as demonstrated by a greater than 40% increase in surgical procedures for urinary incontinence in elderly women, from 1991 to 2001.[5] Therefore, the practicing anesthesiologist can expect to manage ever-greater numbers of geriatric patients in the future.

Outcome studies demonstrate that morbidity and mortality are increased following surgery in the elderly as compared with the younger population.[6] Among the many factors contributing to increased surgical morbidity and mortality,[7] perioperative complications are directly related to poor outcome in the elderly.[8] In a study examining the effect of age on perioperative complications, Polancyzk and colleagues[9] showed

---

This work was partly supported by the NIA grant R01-AG033615 from the National Institutes of Health.

The authors have nothing to disclose.

[a] Department of Anesthesiology, Johns Hopkins Bayview Medical Center, Johns Hopkins Medical Institutions, 4940 Eastern Avenue, A588, Baltimore, MD 21224, USA

[b] Anesthesiology and Critical Care Medicine, Johns Hopkins University School of Medicine, Baltimore, MD, USA

[c] Harvard Medical School, Boston, MA, USA

[d] Department of Anesthesiology, Beth Israel Deaconess Medical School, 330 Brookline Avenue, Boston, MA 02215, USA

* Corresponding author. Department of Anesthesiology, Johns Hopkins Bayview Medical Center, Johns Hopkins Medical Institutions, 4940 Eastern Avenue, A588, Baltimore, MD 21224.

E-mail address: fsieber1@jhmi.edu

Anesthesiology Clin 29 (2011) 83–97

doi:10.1016/j.anclin.2010.11.011

that fatal and major complications increase with age. In addition, perioperative complications in the elderly are associated with greater mortality. Hamel and colleagues[10] showed that patients aged 80 years and older with complications after a major surgery have a 25% greater 30-day mortality than patients without complications. Thus, quality initiatives with great potential for improving surgical outcomes in elderly patients should target the prevention of perioperative complications.[11]

This review outlines evidence-based quality initiatives focused on decreasing postoperative complications in the elderly surgical patient. Of the many types of postoperative complications that may occur in the elderly, neurologic, pulmonary and cardiac morbidity is most common with a reported incidence of 15%, 7%, and 12%, respectively.[12] Because these types of complications form the largest part of postoperative morbidity, this discussion focuses on evidence-based guidelines to prevent neurologic, pulmonary, and cardiovascular complications in the elderly.

NEUROLOGIC COMPLICATIONS

Neurologic complications are the most common type of complication in the geriatric surgical population.[12] Postoperative delirium is the most frequent type of neurologic complication, with an incidence ranging from 15% to 53%, depending on the type of procedure.[13] Other important postoperative neurologic complications in the elderly include stroke and peripheral nerve injury. Because of its overwhelming importance, this discussion focuses on quality initiatives for prevention of delirium.

Delirium Quality Control Initiatives Based on Randomized Controlled Trials

At present, the Cochrane Database has identified only 2 interventions that have definitively demonstrated through randomized clinical trials to prevent delirium in hospitalized patients.[14] One intervention is the use of structured clinical protocols to assist in preventing episodes of delirium. Specialist delirium units that concentrate on the assessment of delirium risk factors and targeted risk factor modification represent a best practice model[15] and should be a mainstay of clinical care. **Table 1** outlines the risk factors specifically targeted with standardized protocols for management, including cognitive impairment, sleep deprivation, immobility, visual and hearing impairment, and dehydration.[15] An alternative to the delirium unit is a combined geriatric-orthopedic approach using proactive geriatric consultation focused on modification of the above-mentioned risk factors. This type of surgical care model was found to decrease delirium incidence in patients with hip fracture by more than one-third.[16]

A second intervention that decreases the severity of postoperative delirium is the prophylactic administration of haloperidol. This strategy has concentrated on patients undergoing orthopedic procedures.[17] Low-dose haloperidol (1.5 mg/d) given prophylactically to elderly patients who underwent hip surgery does not reduce the incidence of postoperative delirium but decreases the severity and duration of the delirium episodes.[18] Use of low-dose prophylactic haloperidol should be considered in vulnerable populations undergoing high-risk procedures.

Delirium Quality Control Initiatives Based on Analysis of Prospective and Retrospective Data Sets

The remainder of the quality initiatives to be discussed focuses on delirium prevention via control and/or elimination of modifiable risk factors. These risk factors for postoperative delirium have been determined via analysis of prospective and retrospective data sets. Except when specifically mentioned in this article, there are no definitive

Table 1 Risk factors for delirium and standardized protocols	
Risk Factor	Standardized Protocol
Cognitive impairment	Orientation protocol: board with names of care team members and day's schedule; communication to reorient to surroundings Therapeutic activities protocol: cognitively stimulating activities thrice daily (eg, discussion of current events or word games)
Sleep deprivation	Nonpharmacologic sleep protocol: at bedtime, warm milk or herbal tea, relaxation tapes or music, and back massage Sleep-enhancement protocol: unit wise noise reduction strategies, and adjust schedules to allow sleep (eg, medications and procedures)
Immobility	Early mobilization protocol: ambulation or active range of motion exercises thrice daily, minimal use of immobilizing equipment
Visual impairment	Vision protocol: visual aids (glasses or magnifying lens) and adaptive equipment (eg, large print books) with daily reinforcement of their use
Hearing impairment	Hearing protocol: portable amplifying devices, earwax removal, and special communication techniques with daily reinforcement of these adaptations
Dehydration	Dehydration protocol: early recognition of dehydration and volume repletion (encourage oral intake of fluids)

Data from Inouye SK, Bogardus ST Jr, Charpentier PA, et al. A multicomponent intervention to prevent delirium in hospitalized older patients. N Engl J Med 1999;340(9):671.

randomized trials that test the effects of risk factor modification on postoperative delirium.

Comorbidities

The 2 most important risk factors associated with postoperative delirium are advanced age and dementia.[19] It is important to systematically evaluate older surgical patients for the possibility of dementia. This assessment identifies patients at high risk for postoperative delirium. Identifying vulnerable individuals allows for the possibility of instituting structured delirium protocols or prophylactic drug administration.

Despite the fact that dementia is closely associated with the onset of postoperative delirium, there is no evidence that many of the drugs used in managing dementia have efficacy in preventing delirium. Donezepil, when given prophylactically, does not decrease delirium incidence in elderly patients undergoing total joint replacement.[20,21] Similar studies with rivastigmine have also reported negative results.[22]

Abnormal preoperative laboratory values (especially level of electrolytes and glucose)[23] and hemoglobin levels less than 10 g/dL[24] have been associated with post-operative delirium. Requirements for postoperative blood transfusion have also been associated with delirium.[24,25] Correction of abnormal preoperative laboratory values is an important intervention in decreasing postoperative delirium. However, whether blood transfusion to increase hemoglobin levels has a significant effect on delirium severity has not been established. Recent evidence from randomized controlled trials suggests that transfusion alone is unlikely to affect the course of delirium in elderly patients with low postoperative hemoglobin levels.[26]

Pain management

Control of postoperative pain is important in preventing delirium. Higher pain scores at rest during the first 3 postoperative days are associated with postoperative delirium in patients undergoing noncardiac surgery.[27] Increased levels of both preoperative and postoperative pain are risk factors for development of postoperative delirium.[28] In the hip fracture population, Morrison and colleagues[29] found that cognitively intact individuals with poorly controlled pain were 9 times more likely to become delirious.

When selecting narcotics for pain management, there is no difference in cognitive outcome when comparing fentanyl, morphine, and hydromorphone.[30] Meperidine is the only narcotic that has been definitively associated with delirium.[31,32] When selecting the mode of administration, there is no difference in cognitive outcome when comparing intravenous with epidural administration of narcotics.[30] There is no evidence that postoperative delirium limits the use of on-demand patient controlled analgesia.[33] However, one prospective case series demonstrated an association between oral opioid administration and decreased risk of developing delirium as compared with an intravenous patient controlled analgesia.[28] To summarize narcotic pain management in populations at risk for delirium, the strongest evidence is in support of avoiding meperidine, and evidence is weaker that mode of administration is an important factor.

Opioids themselves may induce delirium, and elderly patients have increased cerebral sensitivity to opioids.[34] To circumvent these effects, nonopioid analgesics are increasingly used as a part of a multimodal pain management regimen. Several randomized studies have demonstrated that nonopioid-based analgesics decrease postoperative pain and the need for opioids.[35,36] In addition, meta-analysis has demonstrated that nonsteroidal antiinflammatory drugs are associated with a 30% to 50% decrease in opioid consumption and decreased morphine-associated side effects.[37] Given this result, a multimodal approach to pain management using nonsteroidal antiinflammatory agents or other nonopioids allows lower doses of drugs to be used, thus helping to reduce potential side effects.[38]

Sedatives
Sedative medications are iatrogenic risk factors for delirium in patients in the intensive care unit (ICU).[39] The use of opioids is strongly related to the development of ICU delirium.[40] Similarly, benzodiazepines such as lorazepam are an independent risk factor for the transitioning of patients in the ICU into delirium.[41] Among drugs commonly used in anesthetic practice, benzodiazepines[31] have been implicated in the development of delirium. Dexmedetomidine may be the drug of choice for long-term sedation in the ICU because several studies have demonstrated that its use leads to a decreased incidence of ICU delirium.[42,43] To date, there are no studies that demonstrate that dexmedetomidine has similar effects on delirium in the operation room setting.

Medication management
Preoperative drug-related risk factors for delirium include treatment with multiple psychoactive and multiple drugs and alcohol abuse.[13] Drug-related risk factors that may precipitate postoperative delirium include the use of sedatives, narcotics, and/ or anticholinergics; polypharmacy; and alcohol or drug withdrawal.[13] The major psychoactive drugs associated with delirium are sedatives and narcotics, which have been discussed previously. The general consensus is that medications with anticholinergic effects should be avoided[44] because such drugs are associated with increased central effects.[45] Simplification of the medication regimen is important to decrease the possibility of drug interactions involving the central nervous system. A patient's medication profile should be carefully assessed for any drugs that have been associated with delirium in the elderly. Several reviews contain extensive lists of drugs known to provoke delirium.[46,47] The Beers criterion for potentially inappropriate medications in the elderly is also a helpful guide in determining which medications to avoid or eliminate.[48] However, it is important to emphasize that there is

conflicting evidence concerning the potential of many drugs and/or drug classes to provoke delirium (eg, anticholinergics[32]). Therefore, the recommended quality initiatives concerning medication management do not focus on specific drugs. Rather, it is recommended that the patient's medication regimen be simplified as much as possible and regularly assessed for drugs with the potential of precipitating delirium.

Alcohol abuse is a risk factor for postoperative delirium and postoperative cognitive decline.[23,49] Alcohol abuse in the elderly is often underdiagnosed. The prevalence of problem drinking among the elderly is unclear.[50] It is important to try and obtain an accurate history concerning alcohol use from the elderly surgical patient. This information can be used for planning postoperative care such as management of alcohol withdrawal symptoms and helps in determining if the patient will be at high risk for postoperative delirium.

Anesthesia management

Most studies examining elective surgery suggest no difference in postoperative delirium when regional and general anesthesia are compared.[51] Many comparisons have been made among different general anesthetic regimens in terms of delirium prevention. The only positive outcome has been in patients who underwent cardiac surgery in whom administration of 0.5 mg/kg ketamine on induction was associated with decreased incidence of postoperative delirium in comparison to a fentanyl or etomidate anesthetic.[52] However, the results require verification because the study was underpowered (n = 29/group).

Controlling the level of sedation during regional anesthesia prevents delirium in high-risk populations. A recent randomized double-blinded trial examined the question of whether light versus deep sedation can decrease the incidence of postoperative delirium.[53] In elderly patients undergoing hip fracture repair with spinal anesthesia, patients were randomized to receive either light or deep sedation with propofol and followed up postoperation for delirium. The study demonstrated that in this high-risk population, light sedation decreased the incidence of postoperative delirium by 50% compared with deep sedation. The effect was associated with a mean reduction of almost 1 day of delirium for the light sedation group. This study points excessive sedation during the perioperative period as a risk factor for delirium in highly vulnerable populations.

There is no clear consensus as to whether intraoperative hemodynamic management prevents postoperative delirium. Large retrospective analyses of geriatric populations have found no association between intraoperative hypotension or hemodynamic complications and increased delirium incidence.[24] In randomized trials, hypotensive epidural anesthesia in elderly patients is not associated with an increased incidence of postoperative delirium.[54] In contrast, hypotension may play a role in the development of delirium in select subpopulations. Yocum and colleagues[55] demonstrated a relationship between intraoperative hypotension and postoperative cognitive decline in patients with preoperative hypertension. Until further studies are available, no recommendations for hemodynamic management can be made, concerning the prevention of postoperative delirium.

Summary of quality initiatives for delirium prevention in the elderly surgical patient.
1. Structured clinical protocols focused on risk factor modification for delirium management should be used via either specialized delirium units or geriatrician-led patient management. Many of these protocols are contained in the recent National Institute for Health and Clinical Excellence recommendations.[56]
2. Prophylactic use of low-dose haloperidol for delirium in high-risk elderly orthopedic surgical populations should be considered.

3. Older surgical patients should be evaluated for dementia, and a history of alcohol abuse at the time of admission helps identify patients at high risk for postoperative delirium.
4. Correction of abnormal preoperative laboratory values (especially levels of electrolytes and glucose) is important.
5. When using narcotics for pain management, use of meperidine should be avoided.
6. A multimodal approach to pain management helps reduce the potential side effects of narcotics.
7. The patient's medication profile should regularly be assessed for simplification, avoiding polypharmacy and drugs reported to precipitate delirium.
8. Dexmedetomidine may be the drug of choice for long-term sedation in the ICU.
9. During regional anesthesia in high-risk populations, the level of sedation should be monitored and deep sedation avoided.

Cardiopulmonary Considerations

In addition to neurocognitive complications in the elderly, cardiovascular and pulmonary issues present the largest risk to older patients in the postoperative period. The increased morbidity caused by these complications represents a combination of increased incidence of cardiac and pulmonary disease as well as an intrinsic vulnerability due to predictable age-related changes. Turrentine and colleagues[7] examined the American College of Surgeons National Surgical Quality Improvement Program data from their institution from 2002 to 2005 and found that patients older than 80 years had higher morbidity and mortality (51% and 7%, respectively) than all patients (28.0% and 2.3%, respectively) following surgical procedures. Multiple studies have confirmed an excess in mortality and morbidity in older patients, especially following emergency procedures.[57] There are limited data on successful postsurgical quality improvement initiatives specific to the elderly population. There are, however, several strategies to reduce cardiopulmonary complications that are highly applicable to the geriatric population.

PULMONARY COMPLICATIONS

As with other postoperative complications, pulmonary complications following surgery lead to increased morbidity, length of stay, and perioperative mortality in elderly patients.[6] Manku and colleagues[8] also found that older patients with in-hospital postoperative pulmonary and renal complications had increased mortality after hospital discharge, especially in the first 3 months. Although comorbidities predispose patients to postoperative complications, a recent systematic review of the available evidence reported that age remains a significant risk factor for pulmonary complications even after adjusting for the presence of comorbidities.[58,59] When compared with patients younger than 60 years, the risk of a postoperative pulmonary complication is twice as high in patients aged 60 to 69 years and thrice in patients aged 70 to 79 years.[60] Although it is known that older age is associated with an increase in pulmonary complications, there are few trials specifically addressing the reduction of complications in older patients per se, so most recommendations are extrapolated from general adult data.

Pulmonary Quality Initiatives Based on Randomized Controlled Trials and Clinical Guidelines

A rigorous review of available data identified patient-related and procedure-related risk factors for pulmonary complications following noncardiac surgery.[59–61] Patient-related risk factors with good evidence include advanced age, American Society of

Anesthesiologists score greater than 2, congestive heart failure, functional dependency, and chronic obstructive pulmonary disease. The most important procedure-related risk factor with good evidence is the surgical site; unadjusted complication rates were 20% for upper abdominal surgery versus 8% for lower or 14% for any abdominal surgery,[59,60] and abdominal, aortic, and thoracic surgeries carry the highest risk of a perioperative pulmonary complication. Additional procedure-related risks include emergency surgery, duration of procedure exceeding 3 hours, general anesthesia, and multiple transfusions.[59]

The American College of Physicians has compiled several guidelines that provide recommendations on perioperative pulmonary care. The recommendations are applicable to older patients.[58–62]

Pulmonary Risk Factors

Long-acting neuromuscular blockade

One of the few areas in the literature supported by good evidence addresses the administration of long-acting muscle relaxation agents. In a randomized controlled trial, Berg and colleagues[63] compared long-acting with intermediate-acting muscle relaxants in 691 patients undergoing noncardiac surgery. They found that 26% of patients receiving pancuronium versus 5% ($P<.001$) receiving atracurium or vecuronium had residual block. In patients with residual blockade, those who had received pancuronium had a 17% rate of pulmonary complications compared with a 5% rate in patients who had received either atracurium or vecuronium ($P<.02$). Although this trial was not designed to address age-related risk factors, the conclusions are highly relevant to the elderly patient for several reasons.[61,63]

Advanced age is associated with a gradual decrease in chest wall compliance and decreased respiratory muscle strength, so any diminution in strength may lead to hypoventilation and postoperative pulmonary complications. In addition, older patients have blunted responses to hypoxia and hypercapnia, thus respiratory drive is also affected.[64] To conclude, evidence supports that use of long-acting neuromuscular blockers, such as pancuronium, should be avoided in elderly patients.

Intraoperative anesthetic technique

The role of neuraxial anesthesia and analgesia in preventing complications is controversial. There are no good randomized trials specifically for elderly patients, although many older patients are included in most studies. The results of 2 meta-analyses reviewing outcome data in patients receiving general, epidural, or spinal anesthesia found some trends in improved outcomes in the epidural or spinal group.[65,66] However, there are some major issues with the data. First, a large proportion of the surgeries were orthopedic surgeries, which by most criteria are relatively low-risk surgeries for pulmonary complications. Furthermore, the small subject numbers in several studies included and the lack of data regarding intraoperative and medication fluid use make it difficult to reach a conclusion about regional anesthesia. Postoperative analgesia seems to be superior to epidural analgesia for aortic and upper abdominal surgery but has not been shown to reduce the risk of pulmonary complications.[59,61,62]

Lung expansion

Postoperative pain, drowsiness, immobilization, and bed rest are just few of the postoperative events that can lead to shallow breathing and the potential development of atelectasis and subsequent pulmonary complications. Lung expansion modalities include chest physiotherapy, deep breathing exercises, incentive spirometry, and continuous positive airway pressure.[61,64] The goal of these procedures is to increase the postoperative functional residual capacity and expand partially or completely collapsed alveoli. A recent Cochrane meta-analysis included 1160 patients from trials comparing incentive spirometry to no respiratory treatments, physiotherapy, and deep breathing.[67] Sufficient evidence to support the use of incentive spirometry postoperatively was not obtained. In contrast, the American College of Physicians clinical guidelines,[59,61] developed following a systemic review of the literature, support the use of lung expansion modalities including both incentive spirometry and continuous positive airway pressure.[61] The difference in evidence may reflect the methodologies of the review. The Cochrane review only included incentive spirometry, whereas the American College of Physicians guidelines included all modalities. The American College of Physicians reviews suggested that any of the above-mentioned interventions may be superior to no lung expansion, but it is not possible to recommend one particular modality.

Surgery
Surgical site is a significant risk factor for the development of postoperative pulmonary complications, and upper abdominal operation close to the diaphragm is a significant risk factor, with 13% to 33% complications compared with 1% to 16% in lower abdominal surgeries.[58]

Aspiration
Aging is associated with a decrease in the usual protective reflexes in the oropharnyx, predisposing to aspiration. Patients with swallowing disorders, Parkinson disease, and other neurologic syndromes are particularly at high risk.[64] In cases in which the airway is unprotected and in the postoperative period, administration of sedatives should be carefully monitored and strict nil per os (NPO) guidelines adhered to even for minor noninvasive procedures.

Recommendations
1. There is good evidence to recommend avoiding long-acting muscle relaxants.
2. Postoperative pain control: it is not possible to recommend regional versus general anesthesia based on current evidence. However, evidence supports good pain control and epidural analgesia for aortic, vascular, and thoracic surgery.
3. There are conflicting recommendations on lung expansion in the postoperative period. However, given that elderly patients represent a high-risk group, there is probably benefit to providing incentive spirometry or other maneuvers to prevent prolonged atelectasis.
4. Aspiration risk is increased in the elderly and requires vigilant care.

CARDIAC COMPLICATIONS

The presence of cardiac disease increases with advanced age, and the number of older patients undergoing noncardiac surgery is also steadily increasing making appropriate cardiac care of elderly patients extremely relevant. Multiple indices have been developed over years to identify high-risk individuals before surgery. One of the most widely used is the revised cardiac risk index.[68–70] This index identifies 6 independent risk factors that have been correlated with increased cardiac risk: ischemic heart disease, congestive heart failure, cerebral vascular disease, high-risk surgery, preoperative insulin for diabetes, and a creatinine value more than 2 mg/dL. Unlike the risk of pulmonary complications, age has not consistently been found to be an independent predictor of perioperative cardiac risk. However, the intraoperative or perioperative mortality is higher in geriatric versus younger patients in the event of an acute myocardial infarction. The 2009 American College of Cardiology

Foundation/American Heart Association revised guidelines[62,70-72] provide an extensive analysis of the available literature and have been recently revised to address controversial issues surrounding the administration of β-blockers. Several areas are important when considering risk reduction in the elderly patient, including the use of β-blockers and statins, the importance of blood pressure control perioperatively, and the utility of preoperative electrocardiography (ECG). The role of these issues in reducing cardiac complications is discussed briefly.

Cardiac Quality Initiatives Based on Randomized Controlled Trials and Clinical Guidelines

β-blockers

Early data on perioperative β-blocker use resulted in widespread perioperative administration of β-blockers to low-risk and moderate-risk as well as high-risk patients. Data from a more recent randomized controlled trial including more than 8000 patients indicated a reduction in myocardial infarction, coronary revascularization, and atrial fibrillation within 30 days of surgery in the metoprolol versus placebo group. However, a significant increase in death, stroke, and hypotension and bradycardia. These data and others have resulted in a reevaluation of the recommendations on β-blockers use. The most recent guidelines[70,73] recommend (class 1 evidence) that use of β-blockers should be continued during the perioperative period in patients who are already receiving β-blockers preoperatively. Class 2a evidence suggests that β-blockers should be administered to patients with inducible ischemia on testing before high-risk vascular surgery. There is also some evidence to recommend β-blockers for high-risk patients, defined as more than one clinical risk factor, undergoing vascular or intermediate surgery, with careful titration of heart rate and blood pressure. In contrast to the earlier guidelines, β-blockers are not recommended in patients undergoing low-risk surgery. These recommendations are not specific to the elderly but clearly affect a large percentage of vascular patients.

Statins

Statins have been shown to reduce lipid levels, decrease vascular inflammation, and stabilize atherosclerotic plaques. Several trials have demonstrated significant benefits in patients with coronary artery disease, including a reduction in the incidence of myocardial infarction, stroke, and death.[62,71] Recommendations for perioperative statin use are based on observational data and there are limited randomized trials. Current guidelines recommend that patients undergoing vascular surgery be started on statin therapy in advance of surgery, preferably 30 days. Abrupt discontinuation of use of statins has been associated with increased risk of myocardial infarction and death, and thus, continuing statin therapy in the perioperative period is recommended. Statins are not available for intravenous administration. However, there are extended-release formulations (eg, fluvastatin) available that may be used to bridge the NPO status over surgery.

Hypertension

Hypertension is extremely prevalent among the elderly and is associated with increased incidence of coronary artery disease and other comorbidities such as cerebrovascular and renal disease. The perioperative period represents a unique opportunity to evaluate hypertensive therapy, compliance, and efficacy. Every effort should be made to control hypertension preoperatively, and it is also important to avoid abrupt discontinuation of antihypertensive therapy. Despite widespread prevalence of hypertension in the geriatric population, there is no strong evidence that stage 1 or 2 hypertension is consistently associated with increased cardiac risk during surgery.

However, hypertension is associated with increased lability of blood pressure, and intraoperative hypotension has been associated with postoperative myocardial infarction and mortality.[74,75] In a prospective observational study of more than 8000 patients undergoing general, urological, and vascular surgery, Kheterpal and colleagues[74] identified 9 risk predictors for a cardiac adverse event. These predictors were age more than 65 years, body mass index (calculated as the weight in kilograms divided by height in meters squared) greater than 30, emergent surgery, prior cardiac intervention or surgery, active congestive heart failure, cerebrovascular disease, hypertension, operative duration exceeding 3.8 hours, and administration of packed red blood cells intraoperatively. It was also found that high-risk patients experiencing hypotension or tachycardia were more likely to experience a cardiac adverse event.

ECGs

The value of a routine preoperative ECG in elderly patients undergoing noncardiac surgery has been debated. Earlier recommendations included age-based requirements for preoperative ECGs. Although abnormal ECGs are prevalent in the elderly population, abnormal preoperative ECGs have not been predictive of a postoperative event and are no longer recommended universally. Current guidelines (class 1 evidence) state that ECGs are indicated in patients with at least one risk factor, in patients undergoing vascular surgery, and in patients with coronary heart disease, cerebrovascular disease, or peripheral vascular disease, who are undergoing intermediate-risk or high-risk surgery. There is class 2 evidence to support performing preoperative ECG even in patients with no clinical risk factors but who are undergoing vascular surgery and in those with at least one risk factor and undergoing intermediate-risk surgery. In contrast to earlier recommendations, a preoperative ECG is not recommended in asymptomatic patients undergoing low-risk procedures.[71]

Thermoregulation

Perioperative hypothermia has been shown to be a significant cause of postoperative adverse events including poor wound healing, susceptibility to infections, shivering, discomfort, increased cardiovascular stress, and subsequent complications. Numerous age-related physiologic changes predispose the older patient to the development of hypothermia. These changes include impaired central temperature regulation, altered shivering threshold, impaired vasoconstriction, and reduced metabolic activity. Perioperative temperature management is now a recognized Physician Quality Reporting Initiative measure for anesthesiologists.

Summary

1. Risk stratification: the revised cardiac risk index is a useful way to identify patients with increased cardiac risk during surgery as well as an indicator of long-term prognosis.
2. β-Blockers should be administered and their use continued perioperatively in high-risk individuals undergoing intermediate-risk or high-risk surgery, as outlined by the American College of Cardiology Foundation/American Heart Association guidelines. Indiscriminate and widespread use of β-blockers is not recommended.
3. Statin therapy in the perioperative period is indicated in patients with high-risk indices, who are undergoing intermediate-risk and high-risk surgeries. Perioperative statin use should not be abruptly discontinued in the perioperative period.
4. Preoperative ECGs are indicated in patients with cardiac risk factors and active disease, who are undergoing at least intermediate surgery. Age-based criteria for

patients undergoing low-risk surgery are not recommended to guide ordering of preoperative ECGs.
5. Hypertension should be controlled, but limited evidence is available to suggest postponing elective surgery. Observational data suggest that perioperative hypertension and intraoperative hypotension may be associated with increased risk of myocardial infarction and mortality following surgery. Further data analysis in this area is needed.
6. Temperature management is required for older patients, who may require more active warming compared with younger patients.

Process Measures and Quality

Despite the growing popularity of quality measurements in health care, there are few recognized quality measures directed at the elderly surgical population. This insufficiency is at odds with the actual surgical morbidity and mortality data that have repeatedly shown that older patients have increased morbidity and mortality following surgery. The standard quality assessment performance measures for surgery (myocardial infarction, surgical site infection, and deep venous thrombosis) are not specific to the elderly. Although older patients do have a higher incidence of cardiac complications, the same has not been shown for deep venous thrombosis and surgical site infection. The development of more relevant quality improvement methods and markers for elderly surgical patients is needed especially for postoperative pulmonary and urological complications.[6] Markers that examine process are under development.[76] Process measures look at multiple aspects of care, such as interpersonal communication and diagnostic and treatment strategies. It seems possible that these more global markers may provide a relevant method of assessing the quality of care in elderly patients with complications. Using an exhaustive process involving expert review panels, structured interviews, and literature reviews, McGory and colleagues[76] identified 96 perioperative quality candidate indicators of care in 8 domains for elderly surgical patients. These domains include comorbidity assessment, elderly issues, medication usage, patient-provider discussions, intraoperative care, postoperative management, discharge planning, and ambulatory surgery. Within each domain, several quality indicators were identified. In many instances, these indicators are quite specific to the elderly; for example, an assessment of an elderly patient's decision-making capacity and specific discussions about expected functional outcome. This approach provides an opportunity to investigate more elderly specific issues. However, there are significant difficulties in implementing follow-up on such a vast number of both objective and subjective indicators. Despite these challenges, measuring quality of care is especially important, given the excess morbidity and mortality in this growing population.

SUMMARY

Elderly patients represent a significant portion of the patients that anesthesiologists currently take care and will take care in the future. Quality measures and evidence-based strategies to reduce potential complications are present in some areas. However, there are limited geriatric specific data to direct care of the elderly patients. The value of process-based measures is as yet unknown but seems to hold promise for the geriatric patient.

REFERENCES

1. Vaupel JW. Biodemography of human ageing. Nature 2010;464(7288):536–42.

2. Liu SS, Della Valle AG, Besculides MC, et al. Trends in mortality, complications, and demographics for primary hip arthroplasty in the United States. Int Orthop 2009;33(3):643–51.

3. Wang MC, Kreuter W, Wolfla CE, et al. Trends and variations in cervical spine surgery in the United States: medicare beneficiaries, 1992 to 2005. Spine (Phila Pa 1976) 2009;34(9):955–61 [discussion: 962–3].

4. Ciol MA, Deyo RA, Howell E, et al. An assessment of surgery for spinal stenosis: time trends, geographic variations, complications, and reoperations. J Am Geriatr Soc 1996;44(3):285–90.

5. Anger JT, Weinberg AE, Albo ME, et al. Trends in surgical management of stress urinary incontinence among female medicare beneficiaries. Urology 2009;74(2): 283–7.

6. Bentrem DJ, Cohen ME, Hynes DM, et al. Identification of specific quality improvement opportunities for the elderly undergoing gastrointestinal surgery. Arch Surg 2009;144(11):1013–20.

7. Turrentine FE, Wang H, Simpson VB, et al. Surgical risk factors, morbidity, and mortality in elderly patients. J Am Coll Surg 2006;203(6):865–77.

8. Manku K, Bacchetti P, Leung JM. Prognostic significance of postoperative in-hospital complications in elderly patients. I. long-term survival. Anesth Analg 2003;96(2):583–9.

9. Polanczyk CA, Marcantonio E, Goldman L, et al. Impact of age on perioperative complications and length of stay in patients undergoing noncardiac surgery. Ann Intern Med 2001;134(8):637–43.

10. Hamel MB, Henderson WG, Khuri SF, et al. Surgical outcomes for patients aged 80 and older: morbidity and mortality from major noncardiac surgery. J Am Geriatr Soc 2005;53(3):424–9.

11. Story DA. Postoperative complications in elderly patients and their significance for long-term prognosis. Curr Opin Anaesthesiol 2008;21(3):375–9.

12. Liu LL, Leung JM. Predicting adverse postoperative outcomes in patients aged 80 years or older. J Am Geriatr Soc 2000;48(4):405–12.

13. Inouye SK. Delirium in older persons. N Engl J Med 2006;354(11):1157–65.

14. Siddiqi N, Stockdale R, Britton AM, et al. Interventions for preventing delirium in hospitalised patients. Cochrane Database Syst Rev 2007;2:CD005563.

15. Inouye SK, Bogardus ST Jr, Charpentier PA, et al. A multicomponent intervention to prevent delirium in hospitalized older patients. N Engl J Med 1999;340(9):669–76.

16. Marcantonio ER, Flacker JM, Wright RJ, et al. Reducing delirium after hip fracture: a randomized trial. J Am Geriatr Soc 2001;49(5):516–22.

17. Bourne RS, Tahir TA, Borthwick M, et al. Drug treatment of delirium: past, present and future. J Psychosom Res 2008;65(3):273–82.

18. Kalisvaart KJ, de Jonghe JF, Bogaards MJ, et al. Haloperidol prophylaxis for elderly hip-surgery patients at risk for delirium: a randomized placebo-controlled study. J Am Geriatr Soc 2005;53(10):1658–66.

19. Bitsch M, Foss N, Kristensen B, et al. Pathogenesis of and management strategies for postoperative delirium after hip fracture: a review. Acta Orthop Scand 2004;75(4):378–89.

20. Sampson EL, Raven PR, Ndhlovu PN, et al. A randomized, double-blind, placebo-controlled trial of donepezil hydrochloride (aricept) for reducing the incidence of postoperative delirium after elective total hip replacement. Int J Geriatr Psychiatry 2007;22(4):343–9.

21. Liptzin B, Laki A, Garb JL, et al. Donepezil in the prevention and treatment of post-surgical delirium. Am J Geriatr Psychiatry 2005;13(12):1100–6.

22. Gamberini M, Bolliger D, Lurati Buse GA, et al. Rivastigmine for the prevention of postoperative delirium in elderly patients undergoing elective cardiac surgery–a randomized controlled trial. Crit Care Med 2009;37(5):1762–8.

23. Marcantonio ER, Goldman L, Mangione CM, et al. A clinical prediction rule for delirium after elective noncardiac surgery. JAMA 1994;271(2):134–9.

24. Marcantonio ER, Goldman L, Orav EJ, et al. The association of intraoperative factors with the development of postoperative delirium. Am J Med 1998;105(5):380–4.

25. McAlpine JN, Hodgson EJ, Abramowitz S, et al. The incidence and risk factors associated with postoperative delirium in geriatric patients undergoing surgery for suspected gynecologic malignancies. Gynecol Oncol 2008;109(2):296–302.

26. Gruber-Baldini A, Marcantonio ER, Orwig D, et al. FOCUS cognitive ancillary study: randomized clinical trial of blood transfusion thresholds on delirium severity. J Am Geriatr Soc 2010;58(Suppl 1):s86.

27. Lynch EP, Lazor MA, Gellis JE, et al. The impact of postoperative pain on the development of postoperative delirium. Anesth Analg 1998;86(4):781–5.

28. Vaurio LE, Sands LP, Wang Y, et al. Postoperative delirium: the importance of pain and pain management. Anesth Analg 2006;102(4):1267–73.

29. Morrison RS, Magaziner J, Gilbert M, et al. Relationship between pain and opioid analgesics on the development of delirium following hip fracture. J Gerontol A Biol Sci Med Sci 2003;58(1):76–81.

30. Fong HK, Sands LP, Leung JM. The role of postoperative analgesia in delirium and cognitive decline in elderly patients: a systematic review. Anesth Analg 2006;102(4):1255–66.

31. Marcantonio ER, Juarez G, Goldman L, et al. The relationship of postoperative delirium with psychoactive medications. JAMA 1994;272(19):1518–22.

32. Stockl KM, Le L, Zhang S, et al. Clinical and economic outcomes associated with potentially inappropriate prescribing in the elderly. Am J Manag Care 2010;16(1): e1–10.

33. Leung JM, Sands LP, Paul S, et al. Does postoperative delirium limit the use of patient-controlled analgesia in older surgical patients? Anesthesiology 2009; 111(3):625–31.

34. Aubrun F, Marmion F. The elderly patient and postoperative pain treatment. Best Pract Res Clin Anaesthesiol 2007;21(1):109–27.

35. Gilron I, Orr E, Tu D, et al. A randomized, double-blind, controlled trial of perioperative administration of gabapentin, meloxicam and their combination for spontaneous and movement-evoked pain after ambulatory laparoscopic cholecystectomy. Anesth Analg 2009;108(2):623–30.

36. White PF, Sacan O, Tufanogullari B, et al. Effect of short-term postoperative celecoxib administration on patient outcome after outpatient laparoscopic surgery. Can J Anaesth 2007;54(5):342–8.

37. Marret E, Kurdi O, Zufferey P, et al. Effects of nonsteroidal antiinflammatory drugs on patient-controlled analgesia morphine side effects: meta-analysis of randomized controlled trials. Anesthesiology 2005;102(6):124–60.

38. Pereira J, Lawlor P, Vigano A, et al. Equianalgesic dose ratios for opioids. a critical review and proposals for long-term dosing. J Pain Symptom Manage 2001;22(2): 672–87.

39. Pandharipande P, Ely EW. Sedative and analgesic medications: risk factors for delirium and sleep disturbances in the critically ill. Crit Care Clin 2006;22(2): 313–27, vii.

40. Dubois MJ, Bergeron N, Dumont M, et al. Delirium in an intensive care unit: a study of risk factors. Intensive Care Med 2001;27(8):1297–304.

41. Pandharipande P, Shintani A, Peterson J, et al. Lorazepam is an independent risk factor for transitioning to delirium in intensive care unit patients. Anesthesiology 2006;104(1):21–6.
42. Pandharipande PP, Pun BT, Herr DL, et al. Effect of sedation with dexmedetomidine vs lorazepam on acute brain dysfunction in mechanically ventilated patients: the MENDS randomized controlled trial. JAMA 2007;298(22):2644–53.
43. Riker RR, Shehabi Y, Bokesch PM, et al. Dexmedetomidine vs midazolam for sedation of critically ill patients: a randomized trial. JAMA 2009;301(5):489–99.
44. Pratico C, Quattrone D, Lucanto T, et al. Drugs of anesthesia acting on central cholinergic system may cause post-operative cognitive dysfunction and delirium. Med Hypotheses 2005;65(5):972–82.
45. Rudolph JL, Salow MJ, Angelini MC, et al. The anticholinergic risk scale and anticholinergic adverse effects in older persons. Arch Intern Med 2008;168(5): 508–13.
46. Alagiakrishnan K, Wiens CA. An approach to drug induced delirium in the elderly. Postgrad Med J 2004;80(945):388–93.
47. Brown T. Drug-induced delirium. Semin Clin Neuropsychiatry 2000;5(2):113–24.
48. Fick DM, Cooper JW, Wade WE, et al. Updating the beers criteria for potentially inappropriate medication use in older adults: results of a US consensus panel of experts. Arch Intern Med 2003;163(22):2716–24.
49. Hudetz JA, Iqbal Z, Gandhi SD, et al. Postoperative cognitive dysfunction in older patients with a history of alcohol abuse. Anesthesiology 2007;106(3): 423–30.
50. Johnson I. Alcohol problems in old age: a review of recent epidemiological research. Int J Geriatr Psychiatry 2000;15(7):575–81.
51. Bryson GL, Wyand A. Evidence-based clinical update: general anesthesia and the risk of delirium and postoperative cognitive dysfunction. Can J Anaesth 2006;53(7):669–77.
52. Hudetz JA, Patterson KM, Iqbal Z, et al. Ketamine attenuates delirium after cardiac surgery with cardiopulmonary bypass. J Cardiothorac Vasc Anesth 2009;23(5):651–7.
53. Sieber FE, Zakriya KJ, Gottschalk A, et al. Sedation depth during spinal anesthesia and the development of postoperative delirium in elderly patients undergoing hip fracture repair. Mayo Clin Proc 2010;85(1):18–26.
54. Williams-Russo P, Sharrock NE, Mattis S, et al. Randomized trial of hypotensive epidural anesthesia in older adults. Anesthesiology 1999;91(4):926–35.
55. Yocum GT, Gaudet JG, Teverbaugh LA, et al. Neurocognitive performance in hypertensive patients after spine surgery. Anesthesiology 2009;110(2):254–61.
56. Young J, Murthy L, Westby M, et al. Guideline Development Group. Diagnosis, prevention, and management of delirium: summary of NICE guidance. BMJ 2010;341:c3704.
57. Li G, Warner M, Lang BH, et al. Epidemiology of anesthesia-related mortality in the United States, 1999–2005. Anesthesiology 2009;110(4):759–65.
58. Smetana GW. Postoperative pulmonary complications: an update on risk assessment and reduction. Cleve Clin J Med 2009;76(Suppl 4):S60–5.
59. Smetana GW, Conde MV. Preoperative pulmonary update. Clin Geriatr Med 2008; 24(4):607–24, vii.
60. Qaseem A, Snow V, Fitterman N, et al. Risk assessment for and strategies to reduce perioperative pulmonary complications for patients undergoing noncardiothoracic surgery: a guideline from the American College of Physicians. Ann Intern Med 2006;144(8):575–80.

61. Lawrence VA, Cornell JE, Smetana GW. American College of Physicians. Strategies to reduce postoperative pulmonary complications after noncardiothoracic surgery: systematic review for the American College of Physicians. Ann Intern Med 2006;144(8):596–608.
62. Jaffer AK, Smetana GW, Cohn S, et al. Perioperative medicine update. J Gen Intern Med 2009;24(7):863–71.
63. Berg H, Roed J, Viby-Mogensen J, et al. Residual neuromuscular block is a risk factor for postoperative pulmonary complications. A prospective, randomised, and blinded study of postoperative pulmonary complications after atracurium, vecuronium and pancuronium. Acta Anaesthesiol Scand 1997;41(9): 1095–103.
64. Sprung J, Gajic O, Warner DO. Review article: age related alterations in respiratory function - anesthetic considerations. Can J Anaesth 2006;53(12):1244–57.
65. Rodgers A, Walker N, Schug S, et al. Reduction of postoperative mortality and morbidity with epidural or spinal anaesthesia: results from overview of randomised trials. BMJ 2000;321(7275):1–12.
66. Urwin SC, Parker MJ, Griffiths R. General versus regional anaesthesia for hip fracture surgery: a meta-analysis of randomized trials. Br J Anaesth 2000;84(4): 450–5.
67. Guimaraes MM, El Dib R, Smith AF, et al. Incentive spirometry for prevention of postoperative pulmonary complications in upper abdominal surgery. Cochrane Database Syst Rev 2009;3:CD006058.
68. Hoeks SE, op Reimer WJ, van Gestel YR, et al. Preoperative cardiac risk index predicts long-term mortality and health status. Am J Med 2009;122(6):559–65.
69. Poldermans D, Hoeks SE, Feringa HH. Pre-operative risk assessment and risk reduction before surgery. J Am Coll Cardiol 2008;51(20):1913–24.
70. American College of Cardiology Foundation/American Heart Association Task Force on Practice Guidelines, American Society of Echocardiography, American Society of Nuclear Cardiology, et al. 2009 ACCF/AHA focused update on perioperative beta blockade. J Am Coll Cardiol 2009;54(22):2102–28.
71. American College of Cardiology Foundation/American Heart Association Task Force on Practice Guidelines, American Society of Echocardiography, American Society of Nuclear Cardiology, et al. 2009 ACCF/AHA focused update on perioperative beta blockade incorporated into the ACC/AHA 2007 guidelines on perioperative cardiovascular evaluation and care for noncardiac surgery. J Am Coll Cardiol 2009;54(22):e13–118.
72. Fleisher LA, Beckman JA, Brown KA, et al. 2009 ACCF/AHA focused update on perioperative beta blockade incorporated into the ACC/AHA 2007 guidelines on perioperative cardiovascular evaluation and care for noncardiac surgery: a report of the American college of cardiology foundation/American heart association task force on practice guidelines. Circulation 2009;120(21): e169–276.
73. Cohn SL, Smetana GW. Update in perioperative medicine. Ann Intern Med 2007; 147(4):263–70.
74. Kheterpal S, O'Reilly M, Englesbe MJ, et al. Preoperative and intraoperative predictors of cardiac adverse events after general, vascular, and urological surgery. Anesthesiology 2009;110(1):58–66.
75. Bijker JB, van Klei WA, Vergouwe Y, et al. Intraoperative hypotension and 1-year mortality after noncardiac surgery. Anesthesiology 2009;111(6):1217–26.
76. McGory ML, Kao KK, Shekelle PG, et al. Developing quality indicators for elderly surgical patients. Ann Surg 2009;250(2):338–47.

Improving Quality Through Multidisciplinary Education

Rikante Kveraga, MD[a,b,*], Stephanie B. Jones, MD[a,b]

KEYWORDS

- Multidisciplinary education • Team training
- Crisis resource management • Quality • Web-based education
- Anesthesiology

Over the second half of the last century, quality of care in anesthesia improved by leaps and bounds as a result of improved technology and pharmaceutical advances. Since that time, anesthesiology programs have been struggling to make further improvements with minimal success. Attention has been focused on the reduction of human error in patient care because it has been well established that human error is a major cause of patient morbidity and mortality.[1] It is generally accepted that one of the key factors in human error is poor communication between health care providers. As a result, the past 50 years has seen an increase in interest regarding multidisciplinary education (MDE) for health care providers. MDE is perceived as the next means of implementing major improvements in the quality and cost-effectiveness of patient care. In this article, the authors discuss various definitions of MDE, evaluate how MDE might be implemented in clinical arenas relevant to the anesthesiologist, and describe several implementations of MDE within their hospital and the anesthesiology department.

MDE has been a topic of discussion in the medical literature since the middle of the last century. A 1967 opinion piece in a psychiatric journal compared the dysfunctional relationship between doctors and nurses to a bad marriage, leading to discussions focused on the importance of teamwork.[2] In the 1980s, MDE gained relevancy as patient care was pushed out of hospitals into community settings.[3] At present, the increasing complexity and depth of medical training is adding a spark of urgency to the topic as medical professionals attempt to communicate about patient care. To overcome the problems stemming from superspecialization, facilities have begun

[a] Harvard Medical School, Boston, 25 Shattuck Street, MA 02115, USA
[b] Department of Anesthesia, Critical Care and Pain Medicine, Beth Israel Deaconess Medical Center, 1 Deaconess Road, CC 470, Boston, MA 02215, USA
* Corresponding author. Department of Anesthesia, Critical Care and Pain Medicine, Beth Israel Deaconess Medical Center, 330 Brookline Avenue, Feldberg 407, Boston, MA 02215.
E-mail address: rkveraga@bidmc.harvard.edu

Anesthesiology Clin 29 (2011) 99–110
doi:10.1016/j.anclin.2010.11.004
1932-2275/11/$ – see front matter © 2011 Elsevier Inc. All rights reserved.

anesthesiology.theclinics.com

to create health care teams composed of several specialists working together to address patient care. Although this team composition is a move in the right direction, it may exacerbate the problem as specialists struggle to communicate without prior multidisciplinary training.

Anesthesiology is a case in point. Anesthesiologists work with numerous specialists in various fields, including highly specialized physicians and nurses. In addition, their own field has a depth and complexity stemming from patient comorbidities, surgical intricacies, and medical technology. The medical team should be able to communicate seamlessly about the patient without becoming specialists in each others' fields, but this is not the case. The truth is that, although the benefits of MDE in medical school, during residency, and even as a part of continuing medical education (CME) are frequently touted as necessary, although often without concrete supporting evidence, most anesthesiology residency programs do not have MDE as a component in their curricula.

WHAT IS MDE

It is easy to tout the necessity of MDE; however, it is something that has not been clearly defined and therefore difficult to put it into practice. When asked about MDE, medical educators are likely to offer several definitions, each with a slight variation. The terms multidisciplinary, interdisciplinary, multiprofessional, and interprofessional are all terms used interchangeably in the medical literature. One common distinction is that MDE suggests that people from 2 or more specialties learn together, whereas interdisciplinary education additionally implies the goal of promoting cooperative practice.[4] In a 2010 report from the World Health Organization, interprofessional education is defined as occurring "when two or more professions learn about, from and with each other to enable effective collaboration and improve health outcomes."[5]

A definition may create the comfortable illusion of concurrence without providing a basis for uniform implementation. So it is with MDE. Even though there is now general agreement on the definition, this term still encompasses a wide range of educational programs, concepts, and techniques. The level of integration of distinct disciplines in an educational endeavor can vary widely and yet still fall under the umbrella of MDE.

In 1998, Harden[6] published an article that should have shaped future discussions regarding implementations of MDE because it provides the concepts needed to convey the variability within MDE. The investigator broke down the concept of multiprofessional education into a continuum of 11 steps. In the first step, called isolation, the learner is focused on his own profession and is insulated from what is taught in other professions. In the next step, called awareness, educators make learners aware of what is taught in other professions but do not cover this material in their teaching. In the middle of this continuum is a step called sharing in which "two professions plan and implement joint teaching, with interaction between the professions in one part of the course, whereas the remainder of the course has a uniprofessional focus." This continuum proceeds to the final step of transprofessional education, which "is based on the experience of the real world which provides a filter for the students' learning" (**Table 1**).[6]

Harden's 11-step continuum provides an analytical tool to express clearly the level of integration in any particular program of MDE. With his analysis, it seems that the term can no longer be indiscriminately used as an umbrella encompassing a variety of educational techniques without regard to the level of integration. It should be possible to characterize interdisciplinary programs unambiguously in a range from

Table 1
Harden's 11-step continuum of MDE

Level	Name	Description
1	Isolation	Each profession organizes its own teaching and is unaware of what is taught or learned in other professions
2	Awareness	Teachers are aware of what is covered by other professions but no formal contact with regard to conceptualization, planning, or implementation of teaching program
3	Consultation	Consultation about the teaching programs between teachers from different professions
4	Nesting	Aspects relating to the work of other professions are included in otherwise uniprofessional courses
5	Temporal coordination	Timetable arranged so that 2 or more professions can be scheduled for the same learning experience (eg, a lecture with little interaction)
6	Sharing	Two professions plan and implement joint teaching, with interaction between the professions in one part of a course. The remainder of the course has a uniprofessional focus
7	Correlation	Sessions are scheduled in the program for multiprofessional consideration of topics in an otherwise uniprofessional course
8	Complimentary programme	Multiprofessional teaching runs alongside uniprofessional teaching
9	Multiprofessional	The emphasis in the course is on multiprofessional education. Each profession looks at themes from the perspective of its own profession
10	Interprofessional	Each profession looks at the subject from the perspective of its own and other professions
11	Transprofessional	The multiprofessional education is based on the experience of the real world, which provides a filter for the students' learning

Adapted from Harden R. Multiprofessional education: part I—effective multiprofessional education: a three-dimensional perspective. Med Teach 1998;20(5):405; with permission.

those with a very small multidisciplinary component to those with an all-inclusive interdisciplinary approach. And yet, proponents of MDE remain puzzled about how best to provide evidence that MDE is effective.

IS MDE EFFECTIVE

In this day and age of evidence-based medicine, skeptics understandably require scientific proof that MDE is effective before adopting a new educational method. This requirement has proven to be extremely challenging to proponents of MDE for several reasons. Before the advent of the conceptual tools provided by Harden's continuum, any attempt to compare one program of MDE to another was tantamount to comparing apples with oranges. Furthermore, randomized controlled trials of educational techniques have been extremely difficult to design because of human variability in both teachers and learners. Improvement in outcomes can be measured, but often there are so many variables involved, that it is difficult to attribute improvement in outcomes solely to the MDE technique being evaluated. True randomization may be difficult if the control group feels that they are being deprived of improved educational materials or strategies. Without objectively measurable results, MDE seems doomed to experience the life and death of a passing fad.

Despite the obvious challenges inherent in designing studies to assess MDE, attempts are continuously being made to prove its effectiveness. The most recent Cochrane review of MDE in 2009 found a total of 6 studies that were of sufficient quality to be included in their review. Of these studies, some positive outcomes either in professional practice or health care outcomes were observed in 4; however, reviewers felt that they could not make any generalizable conclusions about MDE and its effectiveness. Two reasons given for refusing to draw a conclusion about MDE were the heterogeneity of MDE interventions and a variety of methodological limitations. Regrettably, instead of supporting the value of MDE, such unsuccessful attempts to prove the effectiveness of MDE may serve to undermine the very concept. In reply to one of the skeptics, the Cochrane reviewers stressed that "absence of evidence of effect is not evidence of absence of effect."[7]

Harden serves to introduce a level of objectivity to the evaluation of MDE programs. He redefines the concept of measuring effectiveness in MDE by arguing that the question, "Is MDE effective?" is misguided. In the investigator's opinion, the effectiveness of a program of MDE can be evaluated only in the context of a specific clearly stated goal. If an MDE program is implemented with a specific goal in mind, this goal may be used to evaluate the effectiveness of the curriculum and approach used. Harden's 11-step continuum of MDE provides a framework within which MDE may be implemented, studied, and evaluated objectively.[6]

An example of a study showing a significant beneficial effect of MDE was published by Morey and colleagues.[8] The goal of the study was to improve the collaborative behavior among emergency room personnel. The investigators hypothesized that using a multidisciplinary approach improves teamwork that is critical for maintaining a high quality of care in an acute care setting and possibly also decreases clinical errors. The study was designed as a controlled-before-and-after study. The intervention included both an educational day composed of didactics, practical exercises, and discussions of behaviors and video clips as well as on-the-job training, whereby emergency room personnel formed and provided care as teams while receiving coaching and training on specific team behaviors. Training of all personnel occurred over a 6-month period. A total of 9 hospital emergency departments participated, with 6 receiving the intervention and 3 acting as controls. Observational assessments of the quality of team behaviors occurred at 2 intervals. The study found that there was significant improvement in the quality of team behaviors and a significant reduction in clinical errors that was attributable to the MDE intervention. Of the 6 articles that the 2009 Cochrane review included, this study was the only one that involved an acute care setting similar to the operating room (OR).

On Harden's continuum, this study should be rated as transprofessional or an 11 on the scale because it fully integrates several disciplines into the collaborative goal of providing care as a team. To truly evaluate the effectiveness of transprofessional education, this study should be compared with other studies with the same level of integration of more than one discipline to determine whether this intervention is beneficial. This task is what the Cochrane review investigators found challenging and are thus unable to make a recommendation regarding MDE because the 6 studies evaluated had different levels of integration.

IS MDE NECESSARY IN ANESTHESIA

Anesthesia is unique among medical specialties in that it generally provides a means to achieve a particular medical outcome, rather than being an end in itself. Therefore, anesthesiologists are always working with other specialists and therefore are almost always members of a team. In the OR, these teams are dynamic, with constantly changing players and scenarios.[9] Ultimately, patient safety is critically linked to the smooth functioning of the OR team, of which the anesthesiologist is an integral member. Anesthesiologists working in ORs must be capable of adapting quickly to these changes and furthermore need to be excellent communicators. Excellent anesthesiologists have always had these skills, even though they are not specifically taught in anesthesiology residency.

Recently, more attention has been paid to these skills, even though they historically have not been overtly taught or tested in traditional curricula. This interest has arisen in response to the evidence that most errors in anesthesia are human errors, many of which may be attributed to the lack of certain nontechnical skills among anesthesiologists.[10] In some countries, including the United States, there has been a push to attempt to evaluate anesthesiologists on the basis of these nontechnical skills. A team in Scotland has designed a tool named the Anaesthetists' Non-Technical Skills (ANTS) to evaluate these attributes in the workplace.[11] The categories of skills included in the evaluation tool are task management, team working, situation awareness, and decision making.

Some anesthesiologists are by nature team players and easily adapt to the personnel environment in the OR; they are innately capable of being team players with an acute sensitivity to the situation and capable of task management and decision making; this is certainly not the case with every anesthesiologist. If formal evaluation of nontechnical skills using a tool such as the ANTS becomes a standard practice, training programs will be faced with 2 alternatives: either start selecting anesthesiologists on the basis of their innate ability to be team players or develop a way to teach these skills.

However, these are not skills that are amenable to traditional methods of learning, such as reading articles and book chapters or listening to lectures. Ultimately, to work smoothly as a member of a team, each team member must comprehend the role of every other team member as well as the importance of that role in the overarching goal of providing superior medical care. Once the alternatives are understood, MDE likely becomes the method of choice for training anesthesiologists because it is the most appropriate approach to teaching these nontechnical skills.

HOW CAN MDE BE EFFECTIVELY USED IN ANESTHESIA

Because MDE is such a heterogeneous entity, there are many ways in which it can be used in anesthesia. Again, to be effective, the strategies of MDE as well as the context of learning should be geared toward the goal. In the following sections, 3 different approaches to MDE are described, which have been used in the authors' hospital. The objectives of each of these techniques are very different. In each scenario, the goals of the intervention helped guide the MDE strategy used. For example, a Web module was used to overcome the challenge of having people from different disciplines in the same place at the same time. In the case of obstetrics team training, a tragic patient outcome paved the way for long-term intra- and interdisciplinary behavioral changes in the labor and delivery ward. The orthopedic team provides an example of what Harden would call transprofessional education, whereby a reallife problem is identified and is solved with personnel from different disciplines, and in the process of solving the problem, the personnel are educated about the roles all the team players are performing in the OR.

BARIATRIC SURGERY WEB MODULE

Web-based education can be defined in multiple ways. It can include tutorials that replace live lectures, online discussion groups, or even virtual, intubated, ventilated, and monitored patients. The main benefit of Web-based education is its inherent flexibility. Practitioners can access content at a time and place convenient for them. A variety of materials can be added to appeal to different learning styles and keep the learner engaged-such as multimedia, interactive patient cases, self-assessment tools, and hyperlinks to external sites for reference and supplemental information.[12,13] Interest in a particular topic may be piqued while taking care of a patient, rather than simply availability on a CME course schedule. It is well known that this more goal-directed learning tends to be more effective for the adult learner, thus promoting knowledge acquisition.[14] Web content, unlike a textbook, can be continuously updated to reflect new evidence. Users can return to the Web site at their own convenience to refresh overall knowledge or to seek out a particular answer. Assessment in the form of pre- and posttesting can be easily incorporated into educational modules, which in turn allows for documentation of participation.

Disadvantages[15] include social isolation, perhaps overcome with an online discussion board or chat room, and, in most cases, the lack of ability to truly individualize content, known as adaptive instruction. In contrast, a teacher can alter the presented content to accommodate student needs, interests, and preexisting knowledge base in the classroom or at the bedside. Web-based instruction can also suffer from poor design, most notably when textbook or lecture content is simply dumped verbatim onto the Web platform; up-front costs; and technical difficulties that can discourage the learner. The ideal Web curriculum should have clear objectives and easy navigation and provide feedback.

When examined from the point of view of the Kirkpatrick model of learning evaluation (**Table 2**),[16] Web-based instruction generally leads to learner satisfaction and often to positive learning outcomes. Sullivan and colleagues[17] compared Web-based curriculum training of medicine residents with access to a validated practice guideline on the use of opioids in chronic pain management. The investigators found a greater increase in knowledge and greater self-rated confidence in the Web-trained group. Some have questioned whether positive results such as increase in knowledge and self-rated confidence are simply because of the novelty of the Web-based presentation, and other studies show no difference when comparing Web instruction with other active teaching modes, such as a small group discussion. Nevertheless, the flexibility of Web-based learning cannot be disputed. Burnette and colleagues[18] demonstrated an increased knowledge of pediatric emergency medicine amongst residents and senior medical students rotating through the pediatric emergency department after viewing a required number of online lectures. The investigators felt that this modality was particularly useful in a shift-oriented specialty such as emergency medicine. However, reaching the highest levels of the Kirkpatrick model has been more difficult to demonstrate. Changing behavior or performance improvement has been shown in only a limited number of studies and is usually documented via self-reporting. The pinnacle of medical learning, changing patient outcomes as a direct result of teaching,

Table 2 Kirkpatrick's 4 levels of evaluation	
Level 1	Reactions
Level 2	Learning
Level 3	Behavior
Level 4	Results

Data from Kirkpatrick DL, Kirkpatrick JD. The four levels: an overview. In: Evaluating training programs. 3rd edition. San Francisco: Berrett-Koehler Publishers, Inc; 2006. p. 21–6.

has proven to be difficult, if not impossible, to document thus far in the available literature. For example, Westmoreland and colleagues[19] compared the teaching of 4 specific geriatric medicine topics to medicine residents via the Web- or paper-based modalities. Once again, the Web-based group scored better on knowledge tests; however, there was no difference when clinical application of the knowledge was tested with standardized patients. Therefore, the question of applying this Web-based approach to MDE remains.

In 2006, Drs Daniel B. Jones and Stephanie B. Jones, a bariatric surgeon and an anesthesiologist, respectively, at the Beth Israel Deaconess Medical Center (BIDMC), Boston, were approached by the Controlled Risk Insurance Company/Risk Management Foundation (CRICO/RMF), the education arm of Harvard's malpractice insurance carrier to develop the content for an online module on perioperative care of the patient undergoing bariatric treatment.[20] Bariatric surgery was identified by CRICO as a key risk area after a series of malpractice claims emerged in their coverage area and elsewhere in Massachusetts. Clearly, a multidisciplinary approach to this topic was necessary. The potential complications of bariatric surgery occur throughout the perioperative period. The prevention of and rescue from these events relies on the knowledge and awareness of all involved providers.

Objectives for the course (www.rmfcme.com, bariatric surgery) are clearly stated at the beginning of the module, and a multiple-choice question pretest is given, which is individually targeted to the various provider learning groups. The answers and explanations for the pretest are provided immediately after the test, which helps identify knowledge gaps and engage the student. Flexibility is built into the program, allowing for navigation between the 3 main sections: preoperative, intraoperative, and postoperative, and progress can be saved to return to the module at a later date. However, all parts of the Web module must be completed to access the posttest. Links are incorporated at various points in the program, connecting to items such as a body mass index calculator or the American Society of Anesthesiologists Guidelines for management of the difficult airway. To help keep the course relevant and interesting to the student, patient case examples are distributed throughout the module, which emphasizes key learning objectives. Given the risk management emphasis of this particular course, the cases are based on root cause analyses of actual closed malpractice claims. Users are asked at intervals what might have been done differently to improve patient outcome and decrease liability exposure, given the knowledge acquired within the module. Additional content with extensive illustrations is made available in several "Explore It!" sections. One elaborates on the surgical complications of gastric bypass, such as hemorrhage, small bowel obstruction, and incisional hernia. Some users may learn better from lecture-style content, thus audio segments by experts in the field are interspersed at various points. A reference area containing frequently asked questions and a glossary is accessible on every page, and a "toolbox" provides brief summaries of key concepts. A posttest is given, demonstrating an increase in knowledge on the topic.[20]

It is important to understand how this module serves as an example of MDE. All users have access to all content and are expected to view the content that may not be discipline specific to them. That is, not all topics are directly applicable to all providers, but it allows each to gain an appreciation for areas of risk they may not have previously been aware of. This is a key concept in team training, that is, by developing a shared mental model, providers are empowered to communicate perceived risks to patient care. Completion of the Web module, although done as an individual, provides a means to initiate discussions among all providers in the clinical arena, such as anesthesia, surgery, and nursing. Assumptions of pertinent knowledge or lack thereof can be eliminated from the conversation. Primary care providers thinking about referring their patients for surgery or taking care of them afterwards are also invited to view the module. The pre- and posttests ask different but overlapping sets of questions for the 4 intended audiences: anesthesia, surgery, allied health, and primary care providers. Documentation of both core specialty knowledge (eg, airway management) as well as essential knowledge outside the provider's expertise (eg, long-term surgical complications) can be achieved in this way.

If the bariatric module were assigned a place on Harden's continuum of MDE, a level 7 (correlation) or 8 (complementary program) may at best be reached, depending on how the learner used the information available in the module. For example, if students choose to advance quickly through content that they feel is inapplicable or uninteresting, the MDE aspect of the program is lost. This concern was validated on a recent informal survey of anesthesiology residents and faculty at the BIDMC (Stephanie B. Jones, unpublished data, 2010). Although most survey respondents had completed the module and found it informative, others did not seek out the course despite reminders from departmental leadership. This failure to respond was more common among the attending staff and likely because the completion of the Web module was not specifically enforced. Two residents had informative insights. One stated that the Web module "should not replace teaching from our attending." The module lacks a chat room or other interactive forum, and the lack of human interaction is an inherent and valid weakness. Instructional technology such as an interactive forum should be used to supplement teacher-student interaction by jump-starting the knowledge base and to provide grounds for fertile discussion, but not to eliminate the personal interaction of the teacher-student in the OR. Another resident commented that "surgeons should make it to (the preoperative holding area) early enough to meet with anesthesia and discuss the case." Again, although the Web module may improve the knowledge base regarding areas of concern in the care of the bariatric patient, nothing substitutes for a team discussion before care of the individual patient.

OBSTETRICS TEAM TRAINING

Team training falls to the other end of the MDE spectrum. Almost by definition, students must be physically present and involved with training, not stationed at a remote computer workstation. Team training typically aims to change the behavior of a group on a large scale. On Harden's continuum, most team training projects fall into level 10 (interprofessional) or, if successful, level 11 (transprofessional). Success is certainly not guaranteed. Traditional medical education and the hospital environment tend to breed providers who regard their own opinion as sovereign and enforce a strict physician-nurse hierarchy. These silos of medical care can contribute to the communication issues that team training seeks to resolve. King and colleagues[21] outline several key steps involved in team training initiatives: (1) establish a vision, (2) plan and prepare the environment, (3) train and implement behaviors and expectations, (4) monitor and coach to sustain behaviors, and (5) align and integrate the behaviors. When adapted to high-acuity medical environments, such as the OR or emergency department, team training is often set up using the principles of aviation-derived crew resource management (CRM), renamed crisis resource management in medicine. The key concepts of CRM include appointment of a team leader (event manager), the use of closed-loop communication, frequent global assessment and reassessment of the crisis, and appropriate use of available resources.[22] The application of CRM and team training in medicine is relatively new but well established, and some have been multidisciplinary. Examples include the Multidisciplinary

Obstetric Emergency Scenarios of the St. Bartholomew Hospital and London Simulation; the Team Oriented Medical Simulation at the University of Basel, Switzerland; and MedTeams, a proprietary training program developed by the Dynamic Research Corporation, Boston.[22] These and other programs have been shown to improve teamwork behavior, positive attitudes, and, even in some instances, patient outcomes.[22]

An early example of successful team training occurred at the BIDMC. In November 2000 in the labor and delivery unit at the BIDMC, a combination of medical error, poor coordination of care, and poor teamwork led to loss of a fetus, an emergent hysterectomy, and prolonged stay in the intensive care unit for the patient. The case was well publicized and settled out of court.[23] CRICO/RMF sought a way to prevent such tragic outcomes in the care of future patients. Recognizing once again that communication issues are frequently the driver of clinical errors, CRICO/RMF looked to CRM methodology. The 4 basic modules were developed: communication, situation monitoring, mutual support, and leadership.[24] Each educational module included multiple CRM skills. Team members included obstetric and anesthesia attendings and residents, nurses, and unit coordinators. A new CRM concept was introduced every week or two, preceded by e-mails and communications at team meetings. Coaches were identified, and at least one was assigned per shift to teach new topics and reinforce previously acquired knowledge and behaviors. Positive outcomes and desired behaviors were publicly praised to help sustain momentum and to make sure that all team members were acutely aware of the results of their hard work. After full implementation of the teamwork system, the BIDMC experienced a significant decrease in adverse obstetric events and a decrease in the number of high-severity events identified by the CRICO/RMF and documented a more positive attitude about patient safety among the Labor and Delivery unit staff compared with other areas of the hospital.[24]

Many, if not all, of the changes instituted in 2002 persist today. Team meetings occur at designated times each shift to review patient issues, using templates developed during the rollout period. Each July, entering obstetric and anesthesiology residents attend the 4-hour OB Team Training course, and refresher courses are periodically held for existing staff. Protocols for certain high-risk events, such as shoulder dystocia, were developed to facilitate better team communication. Before operative procedures, a briefing takes place in which the anesthesiologist and obstetric attending along with the nurse caring for the patient review the anesthetic and surgical plans as well as any major medical issues. Adverse events, when they do occur, are actively debriefed.

As illustrated in this example, instituting significant behavioral change via team training is not a small undertaking. This effort was funded by the CRICO/RMF and the US Department of Defense, allowing the coaches to be present in the unit without the burden of clinical responsibilities. The steering committee worked hard to make sure that positive feedback and educational reinforcement occurred frequently. Feedback was actively solicited from participants as well to ensure understanding and acceptance before moving on to the next CRM concept, lengthening the implementation period to longer than 1 year. A similar project at Yale extended to longer than 2 years.[25] The documented improvements in patient care cannot be disputed, and the importance of improved attitude among the staff should not be underestimated.

THE ORTHOPEDIC TEAM

The orthopedic surgeons in the authors' hospital had been trying to determine how to improve the efficiency of their joint replacement surgeries, specifically how to improve processes so that 4 joint replacements could be scheduled per day in 1 OR.

To address this goal, a team of all personnel involved in joint replacement surgery was put together. This team included orthopedic surgeons, anesthesiologists, scrub and circulating nurses, surgical technologists, preoperative holding area nurses, post-anesthesia care unit nurses, and the clinical nursing supervisor who is responsible for scheduling cases and ordering supplies.

Once all the team members were identified, the next big hurdle was scheduling a mutually acceptable time for all these busy people to meet and solve the problem as a unit. One of the biggest challenges to MDE and team training is finding a time when people from diverse disciplines can meet, but it is also one of the essential factors for success.[26] The incoming Chair of the authors' department, Dr Brett Simon, had just negotiated an agreement with the surgeons, nursing staff, and hospital administration to start the ORs 30 minutes late 1 d/wk. Known as "Faculty Hour," this would become dedicated time for faculty development, team training, and subspecialty problem solving. This carved-out time eliminated a major barrier to inter-disciplinary projects, namely the time to meet face-to-face, at regular intervals.

During a 3-month period, this team convened once per week and addressed the long-term goal of 4 joint replacement surgeries per day per OR with an interim goal of finishing 3 joint replacement surgeries by 3 PM. On realizing the significance of the opportunity they had been given, the team then added a second major goal, decrease postoperative infection rates. With these 2 objectives in mind, the team reviewed the entire process of joint replacement surgery from start to finish, from booking the surgery in the surgeon's office to the preadmission testing clinic visit, ordering supplies, checking the patient in, providing antibiotics in a timely manner, preparing the equipment, anesthetizing the patient, completing the surgery, and recovering the patient. At these meetings, every team member present was on an equal footing: depending on others for information outside their area of expertise and in turn capable of providing valuable insight and information to the group. Team members learned about all the other members' responsibilities and the issues that can arise, which may lead to a delay in surgery.

Several process inefficiencies were identified, which are in the process of being resolved. For example, when booking an operative procedure, the surgeon obtains consent in the office, but the consent rarely appeared in the holding area in a timely manner to allow regional blocks to be performed with sedation, which potentially delayed the OR start time. When foreign language interpreters were required, there was often a wait for the busy interpreter to arrive from elsewhere in the hospital. This problem was easily resolved by having portable phones available for conference calls placed to telephonic interpreter services. The team found that because of the extensive amount of surgical equipment required for joint replacement, the circulating nurse had a very large workload between cases that often delayed patient entry into the OR. Now, an additional circulating nurse is present during turnover time to assist.

To achieve the second goal of decreasing infection rates, several interventions were suggested. Timely and appropriate antibiotics must be given. To accomplish this, the holding area nurses were identified as the party most able to ensure appropriate timing of antibiotics, rather than relying on the anesthesia team that may be completing the care of the previous patient in the OR. The team also addressed the suboptimal layout of the OR. After review of work flow and room configuration, the physical layout of the OR was reoriented to minimize the likelihood of contamination by staff members entering and exiting the room.

Throughout this process, as discussions evolved, every member of the team even-tually understood the importance of the tasks performed by every other team member during the course of the day in the OR. Was the MDE project effective or, taking

Harden seriously, let us rephrase the question and ask, "Was the multidisciplinary experience effective in achieving 4 joint replacement surgeries per OR per day?" To date, the jury is still out. As the inefficiencies are slowly resolved, the goal of 3 replacements by 3 PM is more consistently being met. Because infections are rare, it takes more time to realize any potential benefit on that front.

SUMMARY

Anesthesiology has been a leader in patient safety and quality improvement efforts over the past several decades. The advances of anesthesiology as a specialty were touted as a shining example of success in the seminal report from the Institute of Medicine on medical error, *To Err Is Human: Building a Safer Health System*.[1] Yet the prospect of a hospital environment completely free of mishap and mistakes remains elusive. Quality of care can only be improved so much through technological innovation alone because the human factor remains omnipresent.

Communication issues are frequently found to be the root cause of suboptimal care and medical errors. That this fact is understood is apparent in ongoing efforts worldwide to evaluate nontechnical skills in anesthesia trainees, in the incorporation of high-fidelity simulation and CRM into residency and maintenance of certification, and in the breakdown of medical silos with team training and multidisciplinary problem solving. The science of how best to accomplish MDE is evolving, and will continue to change with emerging technology. But only through MDE can each provider understand and begin to appreciate the knowledge and valuable opinions that others bring to the table, whether caring for an individual patient or endeavoring to improve patient care on a system-wide level.

REFERENCES

1. Setting performance standards and expectations for patient safety. In: Kohn LT, Corrigan JM, Donaldson MS, editors. To err is human: building a safer health system. Washington, DC: National Academy Press; 2000. p. 132–54.
2. Zwarenstein M, Reeves S. What's so great about collaboration? BMJ 2000;320: 1022–3.
3. Lavin M, Ruebling I, Banks R, et al. Interdisciplinary health professional education: a historical review. Adv Health Sci Educ Theory Pract 2001;6:25–47.
4. Pirrie A, Hamilton S, Wilson V. Multidisciplinary education: some issues and concerns. Educ Res 1999;41(3):301–14.
5. Framework for action on interprofessional education and collaborative practice. Geneva: World Health Organization; 2010.
6. Harden R. Multiprofessional education: part I—effective multiprofessional education: a three-dimensional perspective. Med Teach 1998;20(5):402–8.
7. Reeves S, Zwarenstein M, Goldman J, et al. Interprofessional education: effects on professional practice and health care outcomes. Cochrane Database Syst Rev 2008;1:CD002213.
8. Morey JC, Simon R, Jay GD, et al. Error reduction and performance improvement in the emergency department through formal teamwork training: evaluation results of the MedTeams project. Health Serv Res 2002;37(6):1553–81.
9. Manser T. Teamwork and patient safety in dynamic domains of healthcare: a review of the literature. Acta Anaesthesiol Scand 2009;53:143–51.
10. Fletcher G, McGeorge P, Flin R, et al. The role of non-technical skills in anaesthesia: a review of current literature. Br J Anaesth 2002;88(3):418–29.

11. Flin R, Patey R, Glavin R, et al. Anaesthetists' non-clinical skills. Br J Anaesth 2010;205(1):38–44.
12. McKimm J, Jollie C, Cantillon P. ABC of learning and teaching: Web based learning. BMJ 2003;326:870–3.
13. Cook D, Dupras D. A practical guide to developing effective web-based learning. J Gen Intern Med 2004;19:698–707.
14. Yi J. Effective ways to foster learning. Performance Improvement 2005;44:34–8.
15. Cook D. Web-based learning: pros, cons and controversies. Clin Med 2007;7: 37–42.
16. Curren V, Fleet L. A review of evaluation outcomes of web-based continuing medical education. Med Educ 2005;39:561–7.
17. Sullivan MD, Gaster B, Russo J, et al. Randomized trial of web-based training about opioid therapy for chronic pain. Clin J Pain 2010;26:512–7.
18. Burnette K, Ramundo M, Stevenson M, et al. Evaluation of a web-based asynchronous pediatric emergency medicine learning tool for residents and medical students. Acad Emerg Med 2009;16:S46–50.
19. Westmoreland GR, Counsell SR, Tu W, et al. Web-based training in geriatrics for medical residents: a randomized controlled trial using standardized patients to assess outcomes. J Am Geriatr Soc 2010;58:1163–9.
20. Jones DB, Jones SB, editors. Risk management foundation web-based CME, bariatric surgery. Available at: http://www.rmfcme.com. Accessed August 25, 2010.
21. King HB, Kohsin B, Salisbury M. Systemwide deployment of medical team training: lessons learned in the Department of Defense. In: Advances in patient safety, vol. 3. Rockville (MD): Agency for Healthcare Research and Quality; 2005. p. 425–35.
22. Sundar E, Sundar S, Pawlowski J, et al. Crew resource management and team training. Anesthesiol Clin 2007;25:283–300.
23. Sachs BP. A 38-year-old woman with fetal loss and hysterectomy. JAMA 2005; 294:833–40.
24. Pratt SD, Mann S, Salisbury M, et al. Impact of CRM-based team training on obstetric outcomes and clinicians' patient safety attitudes. Jt Comm J Qual Patient Saf 2007;33:720–5.
25. Pettker CM, Thung SF, Norwitz ER, et al. Impact of a comprehensive patient safety strategy on obstetric adverse events. Am J Obstet Gynecol 2009;200: 492, e1–8.
26. Salas E, Almeida S, Salisbury M, et al. What are the critical success factors for team training in health care? Jt Comm J Qual Patient Saf 2009;35(8):398–405.

Health Care Quality in End-of-Life Care: Promoting Palliative Care in the Intensive Care Unit

Rebecca Aslakson, MD, MSc*, Peter J. Pronovost, MD, PhD

KEYWORDS

- Health care quality • Palliative care • End-of-life care
- Intensive care unit • Health care quality defects

A CASE STUDY FOR PALLIATIVE CARE IN THE INTENSIVE CARE UNIT

Ms C is a 42-year-old African American woman with a medical history of morbid obesity, hypertension, and 17 years of progressive idiopathic cardiomyopathy. With end-stage congestive heart failure, Ms C receives a left ventricular assist device as a bridge to a heart transplant. Tolerating the device well, Ms C returns home and resumes many of her daily activities. Living with her 10-year-old daughter and regularly visiting her brother and parents, Ms C is on disability, and most of her day revolves around caring for her daughter and cooking and cleaning in her modest apartment. Six months after Ms C is listed for transplant, a donor heart becomes available. Ms C enters the hospital and is taken to the operating room for a heart transplant.

THE BEGINNINGS OF A REVOLUTION IN HEALTH CARE QUALITY

Serious and widespread quality problems exist throughout American medicine. These problems…occur in small and large communities alike, in all parts of the country, and with approximately equal frequency in management care and fee-for-service systems of care. Very large numbers of Americans are harmed as a result.[1]

Funding support: R.A. is salary-supported by a T32 grant from the National Institute of Health. P.J.P. is supported by a K24 grant from the National Institute of Health.
Department of Anesthesiology and Critical Care Medicine, The Johns Hopkins School of Medicine, 600 North Wolfe Street, Meyer 297A, Baltimore, MD 21287, USA
* Corresponding author. Anesthesiology and Critical Care Medicine, The Johns Hopkins Hospital, 600 North Wolfe Street, Meyer 297A, Baltimore, MD 21287–729447.
E-mail address: raslaks1@jhmi.edu

In the late 1990s, this article along with other articles published by the National Cancer Policy Board[2] and the President's Advisory Commission on Consumer Protection and Quality in the Health Care Industry[3] identified a devastating gap in health care quality that many Americans receive inappropriate and inadequate health care. Together with the seminal 2001 Institute of Medicine report (**Box 1**),[4] the articles spurred a decade of intense focus on health care quality in the United States.

The 1998 JAMA article[1] introduced 3 classifications of health care quality defects: overuse, underuse, and misuse. Overuse describes when health care resources are unnecessarily used; in other words, the medical therapy is not evidence based, does not improve outcomes, and fails to benefit patients. Underuse implies a failure to use evidence-based therapy; patients do not receive therapies with proven benefits. Misuse refers to care that is delivered incorrectly; patients receive error-laden care as detailed in the Institute of Medicine report.[5]

END-OF-LIFE CARE IN THE INTENSIVE CARE UNIT—A PRIORITY AREA FOR QUALITY CARE

In 2003, the Institute of Medicine issued a follow-up report highlighting 20 priority areas for improving health care quality[6]; end of life with advanced organ system failure was one of these areas. Patients with advanced organ system failure often encounter end of life in an intensive care unit (ICU), hence an ICU is a pivotal location to study health care quality and introduce interventions to improve quality. One in 5 Medicare patients dies after admission to an ICU, incurring large costs and often suffering needlessly.[7,8]

MS C'S OPERATION

Ms C's operative course included prolonged bypass and cross-clamp times, difficulty separating from cardiopulmonary bypass and the need for an intra-aortic balloon pump, massive fluid and blood product resuscitation, and high doses of vasopressors. Ms C is eventually brought to the ICU sedated, intubated, and ventilated with full ventilator support and inhaled nitric oxide. She is also hemodynamically unstable, requiring multiple high-dose vasopressor infusions. The attending cardiothoracic surgeon and

---

Box 1
Seminal manuscripts in healthcare quality

Chassin MR, Galvin RW, National Roundtable on Health Care Quality. The urgent need to improve health care quality. JAMA 1998;280(11):1000–5.

Hewitt M, Simone JV, editors. Ensuring quality cancer care. Washington, DC: National Academy Press; 1999.

Advisory Commission on Consumer Protection and Quality in the Health Care Industry. Quality first: better health care for all Americans: final report to the President of the United States. Washington, DC: U.S. Government Printing Office; 1998.

Kohn LT, Corrigan JM, Donaldson MS, editors. To err is human: building a safer health system. Washington, DC: National Academy Press; 1999.

Institute of Medicine. Crossing the quality chasm: a new health system for the twenty-first century. Washington, DC: National Academy Press; 2001.

Adams K, Corrigan JM, editors. Priority areas for national action: transforming health care quality. Washington, DC: National Academy Press; 2003.

ICU team speak to Ms C's parents and brother; all agree that Ms C is critically ill and may not survive.

DEATH, DYING PATIENTS, AND THE ICU

More than 20% of deaths in the United States occur after admission to an ICU,[7] and as baby boomers reach the seventh and eighth decade of their life, the percentage is predicted to climb. More patients are admitted to ICUs and they stay longer. As a result, patients are labeled as chronically critically ill if they remain in the ICU longer than 21 days or if they require a tracheostomy because of an inability to wean from the ventilator, although the definition is not yet standardized.[9,10] The in-hospital mortality of chronically critically ill patients ranges between 20% and 50%,[9] and specific studies of surgical patients staying longer in ICUs reveal in-hospital mortalities of 41% to 48%.[11,12] Thus, end-of-life care is an inherent component of ICU care. In the last 30 years, the subspecialty of palliative care has evolved to address end-of-life issues and related concepts, such as minimization of suffering, moral distress of health care providers, and psychosocial support of patients, families, and professional caregivers.

WHAT IS PALLIATIVE CARE

The National Consensus Project for Quality Palliative Care (a coalition between the American Academy of Hospice and Palliative Medicine, the Center to Advance Palliative Care, the Hospice and Palliative Nurses Association, and the National Hospice and Palliative Care Organization) defines palliative care as follows:

> *The goal of palliative care is to prevent and relieve suffering and to support the best possible quality of life for patients and their families, regardless of the stage of the disease or the need for other therapies. Palliative care is both a philosophy of care and an organized, highly structured system for delivering care. Palliative care expands traditional disease-model medical treatments to include the goals of enhancing quality of life for patient and family, optimizing function, helping with decision making, and providing opportunities for personal growth. As such, it can be delivered concurrently with life-prolonging care or as the main focus of care.*
>
> *Palliative care is operationalized through effective management of pain and other distressing symptoms, while incorporating psychosocial and spiritual care with consideration of patient/family needs, preferences, values, beliefs, and culture. Evaluation and treatment should be comprehensive and patient-centered with a focus on the central role of the family unit in decision making. Palliative care affirms life by supporting the patient and family's goals for the future, including their hopes for cure or life-prolongation, as well as their hopes for peace and dignity throughout the course of illness, the dying process, and death. Palliative care aims to guide and assist the patient and family in making decisions that enable them to work toward their goals during whatever time they have remaining. Comprehensive palliative care services often require the expertise of various providers to adequately assess and treat the complex needs of seriously ill patients and their families. Leadership, collaboration, coordination, and communication are key elements for effective integration of these disciplines and services.[13]*

Ultimately, palliative care is a holistic patient-centered care, focusing on intensive symptom management, standardized reassessment of care goals, and concentrated attention to the psychosocial needs of patients and families.[14] Palliative care is not just for the terminally ill or actively dying but rather a philosophy and management plan that explores how a patient understands and experiences his or her illness. Palliative care can be offered not only for a 74-year-old patient with amyotrophic lateral sclerosis, who wishes to forego ventilator support but also for a 25-year-old newly paraplegic trauma patient or for a 64-year-old neurologically impaired patient who has had a stroke. In brief, modern palliative care is about helping patients to understand, accept, treat, and possibly find meaning in the physical, psychological, social, and spiritual aspects of their illness.

Although palliative care, often termed comfort care, was historically differentiated from curative-restorative care, this dichotomy is artificial; quality palliative care easily overlaps with even the most aggressive of curative ICU care. The American Thoracic Society forward a model of "individualized integrated palliative care" for all critically ill patients (**Fig. 1**)[15]; the intensity of curative and palliative care is titrated to the goals and needs of every patient and patient family, and the family receives bereavement support even after the patient's death. A seminal randomized controlled trial evidenced that when compared with curative care alone, early palliative care combined with curative care extended the life of patients with metastatic non–small cell lung cancer.[16] Despite this, both a stigma against and a misunderstanding of palliative care persist in some medical communities,[17–19] preventing optimal delivery of palliative care to patients in the ICU.

Palliative care is, by definition, interdisciplinary care. Palliative care teams must address physical, psychological, social, and spiritual aspects of the illness and thus require experts in all these 4 domains. It is unlikely that any single type of clinician will have expertise in all domains. The National Quality Forum recommends that palliative care and hospice teams include "physicians, nurses, social workers, pharmacists, spiritual care counselors, and others who collaborate with primary health care professionals."[20] The Center to Advance Palliative Care recommends the core interdisciplinary team of a physician, nurse, and social worker with dedicated staff time from bereavement or other staff including pastoral care counselors, patient advocates, pharmacists, anesthesia pain experts, rehabilitation therapists, and psychiatry consultants.[21]

QUALITY DEFECTS AND PALLIATIVE CARE

Although palliative care is desired by patients and their families, it is often poorly administered or more often, not at all administered. Low-quality palliative care can

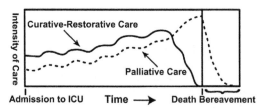

Fig. 1. Individualized integrated model of palliative care in which a patient receives palliative care (*dashed line*) concurrent with curative-restorative care (*solid line*) from the time of admission to the ICU. (*From* Lanken PN, Terry PB, DeLisser HM, et al. An Official American Thoracic Society Clinical Policy Statement: palliative care for patients with respiratory diseases and critical illnesses. Am J Respir Crit Care Med 2008;177:912–27; with permission.)

result in underuse of effective therapies, overuse of aggressive therapies, and misuse of other therapies.

Palliative Care, the ICU, and Overuse

Dying patients too often receive interventions they do not want, failing to improve outcomes.[8,22] Palliative care providers can help prevent overuse by clarifying and reassessing patient goals and wishes and by advocating against unnecessary or unwanted procedures. In randomized controlled trials involving severely ill patients in the ICU, consultation by an ethics team, who identified the patient's known or inferred values, preferences, and acceptable quality of life, decreased the number of days of artificial ventilation, nutrition, and hydration as well as the overall hospital and ICU lengths of stay; all the while, most health care providers, patients, and patient family members were satisfied with the consult, would seek the consult again, and would recommend it to others.[23,24] The use of palliative care consultation in critically ill patients with end-stage dementia decreased hospital and ICU lengths of stay as well as the number of interventions received by patients who were do not resuscitate (DNR).[25] A palliative care intervention decreased the use of vasopressors and ventilators as well as decreased anxiety, depression, and posttraumatic stress disorder scores in family members of dying patients in the ICU.[26] The use of palliative care has also been shown to decrease the number of laboratory and radiological tests as well as the use of ventilators and dialysis.[27]

Of note, none of the aforementioned interventions increased patient mortality; the same number of patients died, but those who did received fewer tests, procedures, and interventions. In addition, patients spent less time in the hospital (2.95[24] and 4.7[25] fewer days) and in the ICU (9.0,[23] 1.44,[24] and 3.3[25] fewer days). These palliative care–related interventions decreased overuse of resources and improved the health care quality.

Palliative Care in the ICU—Preventing Underuse of Effective Therapies

Palliative care decreases overuse of resources in the ICU; the failure to use palliative care leads to underuse of effective therapies. There is strong evidence that interventions promoting palliative care concurrently improve the quality of ICU care. Families note that communication from health care providers is of utmost importance, more important than even physician skill.[28] Palliative care can (1) increase health care provider satisfaction[29,30]; (2) improve the quality, quantity, or content of communication between health care providers and between health care providers and patient families[26,29–34]; and (3) improve consensus between family and health care providers, concerning patient goals of care.[32,33] Palliative care–related interventions benefit patients; despite this fact, many ICUs and hospitals do not offer palliative care services to their patients.

Misuse and Palliative Care in the ICU

Misuse implies that medical care is provided but not provided correctly. Although most clearly exemplified by a medical error, for example, a patient receiving the wrong type or wrong dose of a medication, misuse also occurs when a patient receives undesired care. Hence, it is just as much an error when a patient with DNR status receives cardiopulmonary resuscitation as when a penicillin-allergic patient receives methicillin. Palliative care–related interventions have been shown to increase not only the percentage of patients in the ICU with DNR status[31] but also the number of patients in whom support has been withdrawn.[26] However, despite these increases, palliative care–related interventions have also been shown to decrease the percentage of patients who die in an ICU,[35,36] as well as increase the proportion of patients whose end-of-life care wishes are known and documented at the time of patient death.[36] Palliative care is not about advocating a particular type of care but rather about ensuring that the care provided reflects the goals and wishes of the patient, by which palliative care interventions decrease the misuse of health care resources.

MS C AND THE ICU, PART 1

During her first 2 weeks in the ICU, Ms C remains on high-dose vasopressors and full ventilatory support. She develops acute renal failure and requires continuous venovenous hemodialysis (CVVH). Due in part to the intra-aortic balloon pump, Ms C develops an ischemic left leg and eventually requires an above-the-knee amputation.

Over the next 2 months, Ms C's vasopressor levels decrease but persist. Intermittently conscious, Ms C partially responds to simple commands. She requires full ventilatory support and remains on CVVH. Her critical illness and immunosuppressant medications lead to recurrent episodes of bacterial and fungal sepsis; Ms C's culture samples were positive for methicillin-resistant Staphylococcus aureus and 3 strains of multidrug-resistant Pseudomonas aeruginosa.

PALLIATIVE CARE AND GUIDELINES FOR END-OF-LIFE CARE IN THE ICU

Expert consensus groups, professional societies, and experienced researchers and clinicians have published numerous practice guidelines, consensus statements, and recommendations for both what comprises quality end-of-life care in the ICU and how to measure its impact.[15,37–41] A prominent consensus group, funded by the Robert Wood Johnson Foundation, identified 7 domains of quality end-of-life care for patients in the ICU (**Box 2**).[42] The definition of palliative care, forwarded by the National Consensus Project for Quality Palliative Care, clearly meets these recommendations. Thus, good end-of-life care is palliative care.

Through published end-of-life care recommendations, the American Academy of Critical Care Medicine calls for "family-centered care…[that] emphasizes the importance of the social structure within which patients are embedded."[39] The Academy requires ICU clinicians to be skilled in withdrawing multiple modalities of life-sustaining treatment; facile in using sedatives, analgesics, and nonpharmacologic therapies to

---

Box 2
The 7 domains for quality end-of-life care for patients in the ICU, as identified by the Robert Wood Johnson Foundation consensus group

1. Patient- and family-centered decision making

2. Communication

3. Continuity of care

4. Emotional and practical support of patients and families

5. Symptom management and comfort care

6. Spiritual support

7. Emotional and organizational support for ICU clinicians

Data from Mularski RA, Curtis JR, Billings JA, et al. Proposed quality measures for palliative care in the critically ill: a consensus from the Robert Wood Johnson Foundation Critical Care Workgroup. Crit Care Med 2006;34(Suppl 11):S404–11.

ease patient suffering; and able to compassionately and effectively communicate with patient families. The Academy also recommends bereavement programs for both families and clinical staff. These guidelines are again met through palliative care. The American Thoracic Society specifically recommends palliative care for patients with respiratory disease and critical illness.[15]

MS C AND THE ICU, PART 2

After Ms C has been in the ICU for 3 months, many clinicians think that her case is futile. At the bedside continuously, Ms C's parents maintain hope for a meaningful recovery. Thinking that Ms C's poor mental status is a result of oversedation, Ms C's mother asks that the administration of pain medicines and sedatives be stopped. When a nurse administers a pain medicine, Ms C's mother accuses the nurse of "trying to kill my daughter" and asks the nurse to "leave the room." Eventually, there are only a few nurses assigned to Ms C; others either refuse or have been thrown out. Many of the nurses assigned to Ms C feel moral distress. They are concerned that Ms C has untreated pain and is suffering needlessly. Many are also distraught that her daughter has neither visited nor spoken to her mother since before the surgery. Negative feelings regarding Ms C and her care pervade the ICU; there is low morale amongst the ICU nurses, physicians, social workers, pharmacists, and chaplains.

PALLIATIVE CARE AND MORAL DISTRESS

Burnout and moral distress among ICU clinicians are commonly associated with end-of-life care.[43,44] Moral distress not only causes clinicians to be dissatisfied with their work but also causes them to quit, or consider quitting, their jobs.[45] However, improving collaboration between physicians and nurses can decrease moral distress,[45,46] prevent clinician burnout,[47] and improve patient outcomes.[48,49] Palliative care teams promote these collaborations, facilitate communication between health care providers, and provide bereavement counseling and spiritual support to care providers. In tending to dying patients, palliative care providers also relieve the ICU team from some of that care burden. Thus, palliative care combats health care provider moral distress and burnout.

PALLIATIVE CARE INTERVENTIONS AND THE STUDY TO UNDERSTAND PROGNOSES AND PREFERENCES FOR OUTCOMES AND RISKS OF TREATMENTS

As a seminal trial in end-of-life and advance care planning, the Study to Understand Prognoses and Preferences for Outcomes and Risks of Treatments (SUPPORT)[8] trial deserves special discussion. In the late 1980s and early 1990s, this large, well-powered, multicenter clinical trial evidenced that an advance care planning intervention resulted in no measured changes in the discussions concerning cardiopulmonary resuscitation, timing of DNR orders, physician knowledge of a patient's preferences for end-of-life care, use of hospital resources, and number of days in the ICU before a patient's death. The SUPPORT intervention included daily prognostic information to physicians and a single study nurse to discuss advance directives with patients. The SUPPORT intervention was not palliative care; most prominently, it did not involve a multidisciplinary team. However, the negative results of SUPPORT caused many to think that advance care planning, as well as palliative care, was ineffective.

At the time of the SUPPORT intervention, the health care community's knowledge of how to translate evidence into practice was immature; inadequate evidence of which practices improve end-of-life care and a poor understanding of how to effectively translate evidence into general practice caused researchers, health policy advocates, and general practitioners to fail to appreciate the complex technical and adaptive (emotional, social, political, cultural) barriers inherent in changing clinician behavior.[50,51] Consequently, interventions, such as the SUPPORT intervention, were not designed to overcome these multifaceted barriers. The last decade has ushered in a new understanding into how to change clinician behavior and how to more effectively design palliative care interventions. There are many theories as to why SUPPORT was a negative trial. However, the SUPPORT intervention differs from palliative care, and this difference may explain why, despite the negative results of SUPPORT, other trials of palliative care–related interventions show benefits.

THE DEATH OF MS C

Ethics consultations are called to address both the moral distress of the ICU team and the question of futility of care. A palliative care provider, working with an interdisciplinary team including an advance practice nurse, social worker, pharmacist, and chaplain, concurrently begins to care for Ms C. After detailed discussions, Ms C's pain regiment is liberalized to better address her physical signs of discomfort associated with dressing changes and other painful stimuli. After further discussions, she is also given DNR status. Ms C had expressed a specific wish that she should not be seen "sick and in the hospital" by her daughter. Instead, the palliative care provider liaises with hospital child-life services and the family's local pastor to enable Ms C's daughter to place a telephone call. The telephone receiver is placed next to Ms C's ear, and Ms C's daughter speaks to her mother, including being able to say "good-bye" to her. After multiple further discussions and family meetings, Ms C's family, the ICU team, the palliative care team, and the surgical team agree to withdraw life support; Ms C dies peacefully with her parents and brother at her bedside.

WHO SHOULD PROVIDE PALLIATIVE CARE IN THE ICU

Palliative care is inexorably linked to critical care. Ideally, palliative care should be provided by ICU teams, with complex cases managed by a subspecialty palliative care team. Palliative care is analogous to many other consulting services used by ICU teams. For example, ICU care providers have the knowledge to independently treat ventilator-associated pneumonia but often consult infectious disease specialists in case of a complicated or atypical infection. Ideally, ICU care providers, already an interdisciplinary team composed of nurses, physicians, pharmacists, and social workers, should similarly be able to provide routine palliative care, with subspecialty palliative care providers consulted, as needed.

BARRIERS TO HIGH-QUALITY PALLIATIVE CARE

There are a variety of reasons why palliative care in the ICU is often poor. Some clinicians may lack the knowledge and skills needed to practice palliative care or may find discussing end-of-life issues to be emotionally challenging. Some ICUs may not have a system or the resources to coordinate interdisciplinary family meetings.

Through focus groups, the authors identified logistical barriers, cultural barriers, barriers concerning a perceived lack of education about end-of-life care, and barriers involving care provider refusal to acknowledge that a patient is likely to die. As these barriers are better understood, quality improvement initiatives can begin to overcome the barriers and improve the delivery of palliative and end-of-life care.

There are also economic barriers to providing palliative care. Palliative care is time consuming, requiring clinicians to schedule family meetings and to talk to each other and families. Yet reimbursement for these efforts is poor. The current ICU billing model limits physician reimbursement for discussing end-of-life wishes with patients. In addition, many hospitals do not yet have specialty palliative teams available. There are also political and social barriers to palliative care. Palliative care is hindered by public and policy maker misunderstanding, particularly when it promotes fear regarding rationing of medical care, which is typified by the debates over death panels in the summer of 2009.[52] Thus, even when ICU care providers desire to incorporate more and better palliative care into daily practice, they may not have the time, skill set, or political approval to do so. Further research and public discussion are needed to identify and overcome these barriers.

THE AFTERMATH OF MS C'S DEATH

After Ms C's death, her parents, brother, and daughter are introduced to a bereavement counselor who follows up with them over the next few months. A debriefing meeting is also convened for the ICU and surgical teams; outside facilitators foster a discussion of Ms C's case, including remembrances of her, explorations into the difficulties in caring for her, and explanations into what could be done to prevent similar difficulties in future cases.

SUMMARY

Seminal articles published in the late 1990s[1–6] increased awareness of health care quality and the importance of high-quality end-of-life care. Providing resource-intensive care to the sickest of patients, ICUs are a key place to improve the quality of end-of-life care, and palliative care is emerging as a means. The palliative care–related interventions summarized in this article are heterogeneous. Although the structure of palliative care in an ICU varies by the local context and resources, all hospitals, ICUs, and health care providers need to ensure that patients receive evidence-based palliative care that relieves suffering, improves communication, adheres to patient values and wishes, and occurs alongside—rather than separate from—curative care.

REFERENCES

1. Chassin MR, Galvin RW. The urgent need to improve health care quality. Institute of Medicine National Roundtable on Health Care Quality. JAMA 1998;280(11): 1000–5.
2. Hewitt M, Simone JV, editors. Ensuring quality cancer care. Washington, DC: National Academy Press; 1999.
3. Advisory Commission on Consumer Protection and Quality in the Health Care Industry, editor. Quality first: better health care for all Americans: final report to the president of the United States. Washington, DC: U.S. Government Printing Office; 1998.
4. Institute of Medicine. Crossing the quality chasm: a new health system for the twenty-first century. Washington, DC: National Academy Press; 2001.
5. Kohn LT, Corrigan JM, Donaldson MS, editors. To err is human: building a safer health system. Washington, DC: National Academy Press; 1999.
6. Adams K, Corrigan JM, editors. Priority areas for national action: transforming health care quality. Washington, DC: National Academy Press; 2003.

7. Angus DC, Barnato AE, Linde-Zwirble WT, et al. Use of intensive care at the end of life in the United States: an epidemiologic study. Crit Care Med 2004;32(3): 638–43.

8. A controlled trial to improve care for seriously ill hospitalized patients. The Study to Understand Prognoses and Preferences for Outcomes and Risks of Treatments (SUPPORT). The SUPPORT Principal Investigators. JAMA 1995;274(20):1591–8.

9. Nelson JE, Cox CE, Hope AA, et al. Concise clinical review: chronic critical illness. Am J Respir Crit Care Med 2010;182(4):446–54.

10. Carson SS, Bach PB. The epidemiology and costs of chronic critical illness. Crit Care Clin 2002;18(3):461–76.

11. Lipsett PA, Swoboda SM, Dickerson J, et al. Survival and functional outcome after prolonged intensive care unit stay. Ann Surg 2000;231(2):262–8.

12. Hartl WH, Wolf H, Schneider CP, et al. Acute and long-term survival in chronically critically ill surgical patients: a retrospective observational study. Crit Care 2007; 11(3):R55.

13. National Consensus Project for Quality Palliative Care. Clinical practice guidelines for quality palliative care. 2nd edition. Pittsburgh (PA): National Consensus Project for Quality Palliative Care; 2009. p. 80.

14. Daly BJ. Organizational change and improving the quality of palliative care in the ICU. In: Curtis JR, Rubenfeld GD, editors. Oxford (UK): Oxford University Press; 2001. p. 257.

15. Lanken PN, Terry PB, Delisser HM, et al. An official American Thoracic Society clinical policy statement: palliative care for patients with respiratory diseases and critical illnesses. Am J Respir Crit Care Med 2008;177(8):912–27.

16. Temel JS, Greer JA, Muzikansy A, et al. Early palliative care for patients with metastatic non-small cell lung cancer. N Engl J Med 2010;363:733–42.

17. Cassell J, Buchman TG, Streat S, et al. Surgeons, intensivists, and the covenant of care: administrative models and values affecting care at the end of life – updated [Including commentary by Buchman TG and Stewart RM]. Crit Care Med 2003;31(5):1551–9.

18. Cassell J. Life and death in intensive care. Philadelphia: Temple University Press; 2005.

19. Bradley CT, Brasel KJ. Developing guidelines that identify patients who would benefit from palliative care services in the surgical intensive care unit. Crit Care Med 2009;37(3):946–50.

20. National Quality Forum. A national framework and preferred practices for palliative and hospice care. Washington, DC: National Quality Forum; 2006.

21. Center to Advance Palliative Care. Staffing a palliative care program; 2010. Available at: http://www.capc.org/building-a-hospital-based-palliative-care-program/implementation/staffing. Accessed July 16, 2010.

22. Ahronheim JC, Morrison RS, Baskin SA, et al. Treatment of the dying in the acute care hospital. Advanced dementia and metastatic cancer. Arch Intern Med 1996; 156(18):2094–100.

23. Schneiderman LJ, Gilmer T, Teetzel HD. Impact of ethics consultations in the intensive care setting: a randomized, controlled trial. Crit Care Med 2000; 28(12):3920–4.

24. Schneiderman LJ, Gilmer T, Teetzel HD, et al. Effect of ethics consultations on nonbeneficial life-sustaining treatments in the intensive care setting: a randomized controlled trial. JAMA 2003;290(9):1166–72.

25. Campbell ML, Guzman JA. Impact of a proactive approach to improve end-of-life care in a medical ICU. Chest 2003;123(1):266–71.

26. Lautrette A, Darmon M, Megarbane B, et al. A communication strategy and brochure for relatives of patients dying in the ICU. N Engl J Med 2007;356(5):469–78.

27. O'Mahony S, McHenry J, Blank AE, et al. Preliminary report of the integration of a palliative care team into an intensive care unit. Palliat Med 2010;24(2):154–65.

28. Hanson LC, Danis M, Garrett J. What is wrong with end-of-life care? Opinions of bereaved family members. J Am Geriatr Soc 1997;45(11):1339–44.

29. Treece PD, Engelberg RA, Crowley L, et al. Evaluation of a standardized order form for the withdrawal of life support in the intensive care unit. Crit Care Med 2004;32(5):1141–8.

30. Schuster C, Schell H, Puntillo K. From palliative care principles to practice: improving the active dying process for intensive care unit patients. Crit Care Nurse 2008;28(2):e30–1.

31. Dowdy MD, Robertson C, Bander JA. A study of proactive ethics consultation for critically and terminally ill patients with extended lengths of stay. Crit Care Med 1998;26(2):252–9.

32. Lilly CM, De Meo DL, Sonna LA, et al. An intensive communication intervention for the critically ill. Am J Med 2000;109(6):469–75.

33. Lilly CM, Sonna LA, Haley KJ, et al. Intensive communication: four-year follow-up from a clinical practice study. Crit Care Med 2003;31(Suppl 5):S394–9.

34. McCormick AJ, Engelberg R, Curtis JR. Social workers in palliative care: assessing activities and barriers in the intensive care unit. J Palliat Med 2007;10(4):929–37.

35. Elsayem A, Smith ML, Parmley L, et al. Impact of a palliative care service on in-hospital mortality in a comprehensive cancer center. J Palliat Med 2006;9(4):894–902.

36. Detering KM, Hancock AD, Reade MC, et al. The impact of advance care planning on end of life care in elderly patients: randomised controlled trial. BMJ 2010;340:c1345.

37. Clarke EB, Curtis JR, Luce JM, et al. Quality indicators for end-of-life care in the intensive care unit. Crit Care Med 2003;31(9):2255–62.

38. Mularski RA. Defining and measuring quality palliative and end-of-life care in the intensive care unit. Crit Care Med 2006;34(Suppl 11):S309–16.

39. Truog RD, Campbell ML, Curtis JR, et al. Recommendations for end-of-life care in the intensive care unit: a consensus statement by the American College [corrected] of Critical Care Medicine. Crit Care Med 2008;36(3):953–63.

40. Siegel MD. End-of-life decision making in the ICU. Clin Chest Med 2009;30(1):181–94, x.

41. Davidson JE, Powers K, Hedayat KM, et al. Clinical practice guidelines for support of the family in the patient-centered intensive care unit: American College of Critical Care Medicine Task Force 2004–2005. Crit Care Med 2007;35(2):605–22.

42. Mularski RA, Curtis JR, Billings JA, et al. Proposed quality measures for palliative care in the critically ill: a consensus from the Robert Wood Johnson Foundation Critical Care Workgroup. Crit Care Med 2006;34(Suppl 11):S404–11.

43. Wlody GS. Nursing management and organizational ethics in the intensive care unit. Crit Care Med 2007;35(Suppl 2):S29–35.

44. Pendry PS. Moral distress: recognizing it to retain nurses. Nurs Econ 2007;25(4):217–21.

45. Hamric AB, Blackhall LJ. Nurse-physician perspectives on the care of dying patients in intensive care units: collaboration, moral distress, and ethical climate. Crit Care Med 2007;35(2):422–9.

46. Schmalenberg C, Kramer M. Nurse-physician relationships in hospitals: 20,000 nurses tell their story. Crit Care Nurse 2009;29(1):74–83.

47. Danjoux Meth N, Lawless B, Hawryluck L. Conflicts in the ICU: perspectives of administrators and clinicians. Intensive Care Med 2009;35(12):2068–77.

48. Baggs JG, Schmitt MH, Mushlin AI, et al. Association between nurse-physician collaboration and patient outcomes in three intensive care units. Crit Care Med 1999;27(9):1991–8.

49. Baggs JG, Ryan SA, Phelps CE, et al. The association between interdisciplinary collaboration and patient outcomes in a medical intensive care unit. Heart Lung 1992;21(1):18–24.

50. Bosk CL, Dixon-Woods M, Goeschel CA, et al. Reality check for checklists. Lancet 2009;374(9688):444–5.

51. Pronovost PJ, Berenholtz SM, Needham DM. Translating evidence into practice: a model for large scale knowledge translation. BMJ 2008;337:a1714.

52. McNeil DG. Palliative care extends life, study finds. The New York Times. August 18, 2010:A15.

Quality Assurance and Assessment in Pain Management

Anita Gupta, DO, PharmD*, Michael Ashburn, MD, MPH,
Jane Ballantyne, MD, FRCA

KEYWORDS

- Pain • Quality • Assessment • Satisfaction • Management
- Assurance

In an era of rapid scientific and technological advancement, physicians can no longer be complacent about the quality of the care they are providing. Within the core premise of medicine is a belief that physicians should commit to carefully monitoring the outcomes they achieve. The goal of this monitoring is to obtain data that can guide efforts to improve treatments and outcomes. However, meaningful and systematic efforts to improve care tend to be subrogated to efforts to minimize the rare critical events, such as opioid overdosage, that may lead to poor outcomes. Although the evaluation of such events can play an important role in identifying areas for process improvement, such efforts are often focused on placement of blame, rather than process improvement.

There is significant variability in how health care is provided.[1] Such variability exists between health care systems, from physician to physician, and often within an individual physician's practice. This variation occurs in multiple aspects of health care, including the decision to treat (or not), the decision regarding what treatment to provide, as well as how to go about providing the treatment selected. There are many reasons for which variability in care exists, including the complexity of the care, the relative lack of evidence available to guide decision making, the uncertainty of judgments based on the available data, and human error.

There are several strategies that can be taken to improve patient outcomes, including reducing variation, benchmarking, encouraging continuous innovation, and using performance rewards. The reduction of variation can be accomplished through the development and implementation of clinical pathways and standardized processes for patient care.[2] Benchmarking involves measuring outcomes against

The authors have nothing to disclose.

Pain Medicine and Palliative Care, Penn Pain Medicine, Department of Anesthesiology and Critical Care, University of Pennsylvania, Second Floor Tuttleman Building, 1840 South Street, Philadelphia, PA 19146, USA

* Corresponding author.

E-mail address: Anita.Gupta@uphs.upenn.edu

the most successful programs. Programs that encourage continuous innovation by supporting a culture of accepting new ideas and testing new models of care can lead to the development of innovative solutions to existing problems. Performance rewards can be used for physicians and other members of the health care team to incentivize changes in individual behavior. Successful programs often use several different strategies to improve outcomes.

EVIDENCE-BASED GUIDELINES AND REGISTRIES: OUTCOMES ASSESSMENT AS A MEANS OF QUALITY IMPROVEMENT
Acute Pain

Morphine has been used to relieve pain over many centuries, before even the birth of anesthesia, which made surgery safe and survivable. Morphine continued to be the analgesic of choice for acute and postsurgical pain until well into the twentieth century because alternatives to morphine had not been developed. However, it was realized by clinicians that morphine analgesia could be improved in terms of avoiding its adverse effects, which include respiratory depression, sedation, and slowing of the bowel movement. Alternatives and adjuncts were sought, and multiple trials were conducted, many of which used intramuscularly administered morphine (or other opioid) as the standard by which the newer therapies were judged. These trials included trials of the relatively new class of analgesics, the nonsteroidal antiinflammatory drugs, intravenous opioid by patient-controlled administration (PCA), and epidural analgesia.[3,4] The thought was that acute pain management could be improved using the newer drugs and techniques either as adjuncts or alternatives to intramuscular opioid, both in terms of superior analgesia and adverse effects. Moreover, simple observation suggested that surgical outcome could be improved using multimodal analgesia, particularly when this included epidural analgesia. Several agencies and professional bodies, in the United States and elsewhere, set about developing an evidence base to support a movement toward using evidence-based guidelines to direct practice. One of the earliest of these pain guidelines, *Acute Pain Management: Operative or Medical Procedures and Trauma*, was produced by an expert panel for the US Agency for Healthcare Policy and Research, the precursor to the Agency for Healthcare Research and Quality.[5] All the recommendations were carefully categorized within an evidence hierarchy, identifying recommendations based on expert opinion without supportive evidence at one end of the spectrum and recommendations based on multiple randomized trials, preferably analyzed within a meta-analysis, at the other. Guidelines continue to be produced around the world,[6,7] and evidence synthesis has confirmed the superiority of multimodal analgesia for pain relief and recovery,[8–10] epidurals for superior analgesia and a favorable effect on some surgical outcomes,[11,12] and PCA as a mode of analgesia greatly favored by patients.[13] Much of the work of evaluating and improving acute and postoperative pain management had traditionally been, and remains, in the hands of anesthesiologists, and evidence continues to support their effectiveness in this role.[14,15] However, acute pain services, often anesthesia run, seem to have achieved only modest improvements, with evidence suggesting that acute pain continues to be undermanaged.[16–18]

Evidence-based guidelines purport to improve practice, in this case pain management. Yet, guidelines alone have not been found to markedly alter practice.[17,19] It takes one extra step and that is to ensure that systems are in place to query patients about their pain as a basis for its subsequent treatment. Another limitation of evidence for improving the quality of care is that the best evidence, that is the randomized controlled trial, does not necessarily represent actual practice and, in particular, the true range of patients, morbidities, and idiosyncrasies that are the reality of clinical practice. Trials can be criticized because their findings may not be generalizable, and they may not be powered to identify serious adverse events.[20,21] To overcome these limitations, efforts are now underway to develop registries that can provide feedback about actual daily practice.[22]

A patient registry is "an organized system that uses observational study methods to collect uniform data (clinical and other) to evaluate specified outcomes for a population defined by a particular disease, condition or exposure."[23,24] For example, cancer registries are now well established and often serve the additional function of surveillance, that is, the program not only collects data but also integrates new evidence into public health programs.[25] Such registries perform several functions, including quality improvement, research, cost estimation and allocation, and information consolidation (regional, national, and international).[24] Registries can be as small as single-center databases developed, for example, by the acute pain service at any given hospital and used chiefly for quality assurance,[26-28] or as large as the 3 national and international acute pain registry projects: the Quality Improvement in Postoperative Pain Management (QUIPS), Germany; the Pain-Out, Europe; and the International Pain Registry (IPR), international. These 3 projects are similar in that they are Web based and follow pain-related postoperative outcomes across hospital populations. Efforts are currently underway to integrate these 3 efforts, and a pilot study across developed and developing countries has confirmed the feasibility of collecting and analyzing data and providing useful feedback, even across countries with high– and low–health care resources.[24] The large national and international databases have the capability of identifying hitherto inaccessible information such as gender- and age-related differences in treatment-related outcomes. In conjunction with outcome data collection, the large, international quality improvement projects aim to develop case-based clinical support systems and electronic libraries comprising evidence and guidelines for treating postoperative pain.[24]

Chronic Pain

Improving outcomes by improving processes of care requires significant efforts and the use of an integrated team approach.[29,30] Physician leadership is critical, but nonphysicians also play a vital role in the development and implementation of new processes of care. There is clear evidence that efforts to improve the process of care can lead to improved outcomes of pain management in the outpatient setting.[31] However, efforts to improve outcomes require the investment of time and money, and results are often not demonstrated immediately.

Any effort to improve outcomes starts with the collection of outcomes data. Simply put, if you cannot measure, you cannot manage. Outcomes data come in many forms, including physical outcomes (quality), service outcomes (satisfaction), and cost outcomes. In chronic pain, the most commonly used outcome measure is patient-reported pain intensity. However, other outcome measures include assessments of physical and mental functioning as well as patient satisfaction with the care they are receiving. Clearly, those who pay for health care services are interested in the cost of the care provided relative to the outcome achieved, often with an eye toward the patient's return to meaningful life, including work or its equivalent.

Previous investigators have provided a broad overview of specific outcome measures that can be included in the conduct of analgesic clinical trials,[32] and these reports provide useful information that can be used to select specific outcome measures to monitor pain practice outcomes. A list of outcome measurement tools included in the University of Pennsylvania pain outcome measurement project is included in **Table 1**. Although the decision regarding specific outcome measurement tools is important, it is even more important to develop and implement a process for data collection, regardless of the specific tools initially selected.

Core outcome measures include patient-reported pain intensity, global impression of change, an assessment of mood via the Patient Health Questionnaire, and a global assessment of physical functioning. In addition, the program periodically obtains more detailed outcome data through the use of measures of health-related quality of life.[33] The Short Form 36 and the Treatment Outcomes in Pain Survey[34] are examples of validated health-related quality-of-life measurement instruments.

The challenges associated with the collection of outcomes in the chronic pain population are not trivial, and few chronic pain programs have successfully developed and implemented an outcomes data collection process. However, there are a growing number of options, often through electronic data capture via hand-held tablets or computers, sometimes supported by the use of Internet-based outcomes data collection.[35] Such systems have been demonstrated to be effective in obtaining outcomes data in a large proportion of the patients receiving care and are well accepted by patients as well as clinicians.

Once data collection has started, several opportunities to improve the process of care present themselves. Care should be taken to select a specific project that is

Table 1
Pain outcomes data collected at the Penn Pain Medicine Center

Time Point	Outcomes Data Collected	Comments
Baseline	• Modified TOPS • Average, least, and worst pain via the 11-point categorical scale • PHQ-9 • ORT • Physical functioning via the 11-point categorical scale	Outcomes data are collected either remotely via the Internet or via computer when the patient arrives. Reports are printed and available at the time of the visit. The PHQ-9, ORT, pain intensity score, and functioning scores are entered into the patient's electronic medical record and used to guide individual patient care
1, 3, and 6 mo, then every 6 mo	• Follow-up TOPS • Average, least, and worst pain via the 11-point categorical scale • Pain relief • Global impression of change • PHQ-9 • Physical functioning	The follow-up TOPS has the demographic questions included in the TOPS removed because these questions do not need to be asked again
All other visits	• Pain intensity • Pain relief • Global impression of change • PHQ-9 • Physical functioning	

Abbreviations: ORT, Opioid Risk Tool; PHQ-9, Patient Health Questionairre-9; TOPS, Treatment Outcomes in Pain Survey.

achievable and for which the results of quality improvement effort can be determined with available data. Although there are limited data to document that such a process can be effectively used in the population with chronic pain, there is reason to believe that such efforts lead to improved outcomes.

Cancer Pain and Palliative Care

Major problems in palliative care are underrecognition, underdiagnosis, and thus undertreatment of patients with significant distress, ranging from existential anguish to anxiety, pain, and depression. For at least half of those dying from cancer, most of them elderly and many vulnerable, death entails a spectrum of symptoms, including pain, labored breathing, distress, nausea, confusion, and other physical and psychological conditions that go untreated or undertreated and vastly diminish the quality of their remaining days.[36,37]

In the early 1980s, the World Health Organization (WHO) Cancer Unit began the development of a global initiative to advocate for pain relief, that is, to improve the quality of pain care and opioid availability worldwide. The WHO developed a critical guideline for pain management, which remains the single most important quality improvement process for the management of cancer as well as pain management in general. The analgesic ladder systematically provides global education on logical approach to pain by describing a 3-step ladder approach to pharmacotherapy for pain. The publication of guidelines in a wide variety of languages has had a great effect on influencing the development of pain and symptom relief worldwide and, in addition, has had a profound effect on improving the quality of palliative care.

To address gaps in the WHO cancer pain guidelines, Seow and colleagues[38] implemented a framework for evaluating quality of cancer care at the end of life. Implementing quality indicators that are reflective of the scope of care, feasible to implement, and supported by evidence may help to identify areas and settings most in need of improvement. To help advance quality indicator development and implementation in this area, Seow and colleagues developed a conceptual framework based on previous related initiatives, updated reviews of end-of-life cancer quality indicators and relevant data sources, and expert input. The framework describes 5 steps for developing and assessing a quality indicator for end-of-life care, defining the (1) population of focus, (2) broad quality domains, (3) specific target areas, (4) steps of the care process, and (5) evaluation criteria for quality indicators. By using this conceptual framework, indicator developers, researchers, and policymakers may be able to refine and implement indicator sets to effectively evaluate and improve care at the end of life.[38] Using this framework, clinicians may be able to more consistently and effectively measure and improve the quality of cancer end-of-life care. Dy and colleagues[39] described the current evidence for key standards in cancer pain management through a process of topic development, systematic literature review, and an expert panel consensus rating process. These included, for general cancer pain, the domains of screening, assessment, treatment, and follow-up; a topic on treatment options for bone metastases; and domains for diagnosis, treatment, and follow-up in spinal cord compression. Dy and colleagues determined that, in general, evidence from clinical studies was strongest for treatment and domains such as screening and follow-up were based on practice guidelines and expert consensus.

The current inadequacy of palliative and end-of-life care springs not from a single cause or sector of society but from institutional and economic barriers, lack of information about what can be achieved, lack of training and education of health care professionals, and inadequate public sector investment in research to improve the situation. This inadequacy is not to suggest that there is no ongoing research on relevant questions or training programs but that the efforts are not coordinated and there is no locus for these activities in any federal agency. What has resulted is underfunding, a lack of appropriate training, and a lack of research leadership, with no sustained programs for developing and disseminating palliative treatments. Despite the enormous health care expenditures for the dying, less than 1% of the National Cancer Institute budget is spent on symptom control, palliative care, or end-of-life research or training.

Several practical barriers remain before implementing end-of-life cancer care quality indicators. Identifying the relevant population is demanding, in part, owing to the difficulties in predicting the end-of-life period, thus leading to difficulty in developing evidence-based guidelines for patients with cancer pain. Other barriers include limited data sources, especially where indicators depend on precise documentation of issues such as communication, patient-reported outcomes, or preferences. Many indicators depend on onerous medical record abstraction. Some indicator sets are retrospective from the time of death, which limits their use prospectively or in settings where this information may not be clearly accessible. Initiatives such as electronic health records can be implemented and prepared to facilitate the needed documentation and collate information on quality indicators. Also, indicators that work well in one setting may not in others as a result of differences in populations or systems, and supporting evidence may not translate across various settings. Many indicators are currently available, but much more coordination, rigorous evaluation, and further development and supporting evidence are needed to evolve the field and make end-of-life indicators a customary part of measuring the quality of cancer care. By using a theoretical framework as proposed by Seow and colleagues[38] and Dy and colleagues,[39] indicator developers can continue to work toward building indicators that are scientifically acceptable and that reflect the scope of cancer end-of-life care, expanding the evidence to support their use and refining effective and efficient ways to use indicators to evaluate and advance care at the end of life. Future research will need to prioritize and further develop the most important quality indicators by setting, population, or clinical circumstance.

ENSURING PAIN IS MANAGED THROUGH A QUALITY ASSURANCE MANDATE

Relieving pain could be seen as central to medical care, yet it is known that pain can easily be overlooked in the present frenetic health care environment. One could ask why it ever became necessary to lobby for pain relief, and although the reasons are complex, one simple factor runs through all undertreatment of pain, unless it is sought, pain can be silent. Unless pain is actively assessed, many, indeed most, patients will suffer in silence. Pain assessment then is the fundamental activity by which pain can be relieved. It is no coincidence that when the Joint Commission for the Accreditation of Healthcare Organizations (JCAHO) adopted pain management as a quality metric for health care facilities, the need to assess pain was the primary requirement of its mandate. Five elements were established, which were considered essential to improve institutional accountability for the assessment and treatment of pain[40]:

- Pain must be recognized and treated promptly.
- Information about analgesics should be readily available to clinicians in a way that facilitates order writing and interpretation of orders.
- Patients must be assured of attentive pain care.
- Explicit policies should be developed for the use of advanced analgesic technologies.
- Processes and outcomes should be examined for continued improvement.

The idea was to make pain management a priority in the health care system and to establish systems to support, reinforce, and reward good pain management practice. The standards were approved in 1999 and formally introduced into the accreditation process in 2001.[41] Perhaps the most obvious manifestation of the mandate was the introduction of pain as a fifth vital sign. Although it was never the intention of the JCAHO that the fifth vital sign should become the focus of its pain mandate, nevertheless it has become its hallmark.

PATIENT-CENTERED OUTCOMES

Pain is one of the few outcomes of medical care, which is truly subjective, another being patient satisfaction. Perhaps not surprisingly, because the pain-free state is highly desirable, pain and patient satisfaction are closely linked.[42] Patients rating of medical care or a medical intervention is higher if associated pain is minimized. Moreover, when evaluating care overall, as in marketing surveillance, a good pain experience is consistently found to correlate with global satisfaction.[43] However, satisfaction with pain care is not necessarily related to the achievement of clinically meaningful reductions in pain scores or, even in the case of chronic pain, improvement in the quality of life or function. This apparent paradox is a finding of multiple studies.[44–47] What seems to matter to patients is that their pain is recognized, evaluated thoughtfully, and treated carefully, in other words that they are not isolated by pain and that they have some control in its treatment.[42,48,49]

The present discussion is not complete without mentioning the difficult issue of accommodating both patients' desire to be pain free and clinicians concerns about the adverse effect of pain treatment. The greatest concern centers on the use of opioids, which although being the only systemic analgesics capable of relieving severe pain (at least acutely), are also capable of doing great harm. Opioids are not only respiratory depressants and potentially lethal (a concern particularly during acute pain management)[50] but also addictive (a concern during chronic pain management).[51] Thus the ideal, that patients should have complete control and autonomy over their pain management,[52–54] the control they have grown to expect with other aspects of their health care (at least in the United States), cannot be achieved in the case of pain management. Of course there is much debate about the degree to which patient choice in pain management should be respected, and this debate is not likely to ever be completely settled. Several problems arise in the case of opioids and patients rights to receive or demand opioids. As evidence-based medicine has developed and evolved, patient choices increasingly become incorporated into the process of outcomes assessment.[55] Patients are routinely included in expert panels as trials are developed, research is approved by institutional review boards, and guidelines are written. Clinicians are increasingly empowered, therefore, to advise patients within a cooperative relationship on the basis of evidence synthesis that has already incorporated patient choice. Confidence in some measures of patient choice, notably patient satisfaction, is reduced, particularly when understanding that patient satisfaction instruments have many limitations and can produce misleading results.[56–59] The difficulty comes chiefly when the patient and the clinician do not agree on a treatment decision. Clinicians' primary duty is their patients[60] but can they completely ignore costs to the society, such as growth in misuse, abuse and related deaths,[61–63] or the growing body of evidence that suggests that long-term opioid use does not achieve treatment goals, at least not on a population basis?[45,64,65] Should clinicians be pressured into providing medical treatment, in this case prescribing opioids, against their best clinical judgment either because of a patient's demand or because they need to meet patient satisfaction and other quality metrics? These questions present clinicians with some of the most difficult and insoluble ethical dilemmas in medical practice.[66,67]

SUMMARY

Relief from pain is itself a marker of high-quality medical care. Whether the case is that a patient suffers injury, undergoes surgery, develops a painful illness, or suffers chronic pain, the medical intervention that results in relief of pain is rated highly, at least by patients themselves. Quality assurance in the case of pain management could simply mean successful elimination of pain. Because the means of controlling pain are imperfect, so in addition to considering whether pain interventions actually achieve the primary goal of pain relief, it must also be considered whether they are safe, cost-effective, and even capable of producing secondary benefits such as early recovery from surgery. Quality assurance and assessment in pain management therefore becomes a complex undertaking that must incorporate into its processes the often-conflicting goals of comfort versus safety versus patients' rights. Thus although the WHO cancer pain initiative was successful in promulgating a simple and effective scheme for treating advanced pain, it has encouraged physicians to provide pain relief to those with intense suffering. The JCAHO pain mandate was successful in encouraging pain assessment and treatment across all patient groups within the US health care institutions. Quality assurance mechanisms must remain active and focused on ensuring that pain interventions achieve their goals. The continued process of quality assurance in pain management has tended to evolve differently in the 3 areas of acute, chronic, and cancer pain management. Perhaps this is inevitable because the desired outcome of pain therapy in these 3 groups differs, for acute being rapid recovery and functional restoration, for chronic being improved quality of life, and for cancer at the end of life being comfort.

REFERENCES

1. Swensen SJ, Meyer GS, Nelson EC, et al. Cottage industry to postindustrial care—the revolution in health care delivery. N Engl J Med 2010;362(5):e12.
2. James BC, Hammond ME. The challenge of variation in medical practice. Arch Pathol Lab Med 2000;124(7):1001–3.
3. Ballantyne JC, Chalmers TC, Dear KB, et al. Qualitative analysis of drug interventions: adult postoperative and trauma patients. In: US Department of Health and Human Services, editor. Acute pain management: guideline technical report. Rockville (MD): Agency of Health Care Policy and Research; 1995. p. 28–106.
4. Ashburn MA, Ballantyne JC. Optimal postoperative analgesia. In: Fleisher L, editor. Evidence based practice of anesthesia. 2nd edition. Philadelphia (PA): Elsevier; 2009. p. 485–92.
5. Carr DB, Jacox AK, Chapman CR, et al. Acute pain management: operative or medical procedures and trauma. Clinical Practice Guideline. AHCPR Pub No 92–0032. Rockville (MD): Agency for Health Care Policy and Research, Public Health Service, US Department of Health and Human Services; 1992.
6. American Society of Anesthesiologists Task Force on Acute Pain Management. Practice guidelines for acute pain management in the perioperative setting: an updated report by the American Society of Anesthesiologists Task Force on Acute Pain Management. Anesthesiology 2004;100(6):1573–81.

7. Gordon DB, Dahl JL, Miaskowski C, et al. American pain society recommendations for improving the quality of acute and cancer pain management: American Pain Society Quality of Care Task Force. Arch Intern Med 2005;165(14):1574–80.
8. Kehlet H, Dahl JB. Anaesthesia, surgery, and challenges in postoperative recovery. Lancet 2003;362(9399):1921–8.
9. Elia N, Lysakowski C, Tramer MR. Does multimodal analgesia with acetaminophen, nonsteroidal antiinflammatory drugs, or selective cyclooxygenase-2 inhibitors and patient-controlled analgesia morphine offer advantages over morphine alone? Meta-analyses of randomized trials. Anesthesiology 2005;103(6):1296–304.
10. White PF, Kehlet H, Neal JM, et al. The role of the anesthesiologist in fast-track surgery: from multimodal analgesia to perioperative medical care. Anesth Analg 2007;104(6):1380–96.
11. Ballantyne JC. Does epidural analgesia improve surgical outcome? Br J Anaesth 2004;92(1):4–6.
12. Ballantyne JC, Kupelnick B, McPeek B, et al. Does the evidence support the use of spinal and epidural anesthesia for surgery? J Clin Anesth 2005;17(5):382–91.
13. Walder B, Schafer M, Henzi I, et al. Efficacy and safety of patient-controlled opioid analgesia for acute postoperative pain: a quantitative systematic review. Acta Anaesthesiol Scand 2001;45(7):795–804.
14. Miaskowski C, Crews J, Ready LB, et al. Anesthesia-based pain services improve the quality of postoperative pain management. Pain 1999;80(1–2):23–9.
15. Warfield CA, Kahn CH. Acute pain management: programs in the US hospitals and experiences and attitudes among US adults. Anesthesiology 1995;83(5):1090–4.
16. Rawal N. Acute pain services revisited—good from far, far from good? Reg Anesth Pain Med 2002;27(2):117–21.
17. Apfelbaum JL, Chen C, Mehta SS, et al. Postoperative pain experience: results from a national survey suggest postoperative pain continues to be undermanaged. Anesth Analg 2003;97(2):534–40.
18. Stomberg MW, Wickstrom K, Joelsson H, et al. Postoperative pain management on surgical wards—do quality assurance strategies result in long-term effects on staff member attitudes and clinical outcomes? Pain Manag Nurs 2003; 4(1):11–22.
19. Gordon DB, Dahl JL. Quality improvement challenges in pain management. Pain 2004;107(1–2):1–4.
20. Liu SS, Warren DT, Wu CL, et al. A lovely idea: forming an ASRA Acute Postoperative Pain (AcutePOP) database. Reg Anesth Pain Med 2006;31(4):291–3.
21. McQuay H, Moore A. Utility of clinical trial results for clinical practice. Eur J Pain 2007;11(2):123–4.
22. Parkin DM. The evolution of the population-based cancer registry. Nat Rev Cancer 2006;6(8):603–12.
23. Gliklich RE, Dreyer NA, editors. Registries for evaluating patient outcomes: a user's guide. Rockville (MD): Agency for Healthcare Research and Quality; 2007. p. 163–82.
24. Zaslansky R, Chapman R, Meissner W. Registries for acute pain: will they advance evidence-based practice? APS Bulletin 2009;19(2):6–9. Available at: http://www.ampainsoc.org/pub/bulletin/sum09/innovations.htm. Accessed July 1, 2010.
25. Parkin DM. The role of cancer registries in cancer control. Int J Clin Oncol 2008; 13(2):102–11.
26. Ballantyne JC, McKenna JM, Ryder E. Epidural analgesia—experience of 5628 patients in a large teaching hospital derived through audit. Acute Pain 2003;4: 89–97.

27. Cheung CW, Ying CL, Lee LH, et al. An audit of postoperative intravenous patient-controlled analgesia with morphine: evolution over the last decade. Eur J Pain 2009;13(5):464–71.

28. Popping DM, Zahn PK, Van Aken HK, et al. Effectiveness and safety of postoperative pain management: a survey of 18925 consecutive patients between 1998 and 2006 (2nd revision): a database analysis of prospectively raised data. Br J Anaesth 2008;101(6):832–40.

29. Steele JR, Wallace MJ, Hovsepian DM, et al. Guidelines for establishing a quality improvement program in interventional radiology. J Vasc Interv Radiol 2010;21(5):617–25.

30. Pauker SG, Zane EM, Salem DN. Creating a safer health care system: finding the constraint. JAMA 2005;294(22):2906–8.

31. Magill MK, Day J, Mervis A, et al. Improving colonoscopy referral rates through computer-supported, primary care practice redesign. J Healthc Qual 2009;31(4):43–52 [quiz: 52–3].

32. Turk DC, Dworkin RH, Allen RR, et al. Core outcome domains for chronic pain clinical trials: IMMPACT recommendations. Pain 2003;106(3):337–45.

33. Vetter TR. A primer on health-related quality of life in chronic pain medicine. Anesth Analg 2007;104(3):703–18.

34. Rogers WH, Wittink HM, Ashburn MA, et al. Using the "TOPS," an outcomes instrument for multidisciplinary outpatient pain treatment. Pain Med 2000;1(1):55–67.

35. Podichetty VK, Weiss LT, Fanciullo GJ, et al. Web-based health survey systems in outcome assessment and management of pain. Pain Med 2007;8(Suppl 3):S189–98.

36. Donnelly S, Walsh D, Rybicki L. The symptoms of advanced cancer: identification of clinical and research priorities by assessment of prevalence and severity. J Palliat Care 1995;11(1):27–32.

37. Phillips DF. End-of-life coalitions grow to fill needs. JAMA 2000;284(19):2442–4.

38. Seow H, Snyder CF, Mularski RA, et al. A framework for assessing quality indicators for cancer care at the end of life. J Pain Symptom Manage 2009;38(6):903–12.

39. Dy SM, Asch SM, Naeim A, et al. Evidence-based standards for cancer pain management. J Clin Oncol 2008;26(23):3879–85.

40. Dahl JL, Gordon DB. Joint Commission pain standards: a progress report. APS Bulletin 2002;12(6):1–8.

41. Joint Commission on Accreditation of Healthcare Organizations pain management standards. 2001. Effective January 1, 2001. Available at: http://www.jcaho.org/standard/. Accessed July 1, 2010.

42. Comley AL, DeMeyer E. Assessing patient satisfaction with pain management through a continuous quality improvement effort. J Pain Symptom Manage 2001;21(1):27–40.

43. Wu CL, Naqibuddin M, Fleisher LA. Measurement of patient satisfaction as an outcome of regional anesthesia and analgesia: a systematic review. Reg Anesth Pain Med 2001;26:196–208.

44. Ward SE, Gordon DB. Patient satisfaction and pain severity as outcomes in pain management: a longitudinal view of one setting's experience. J Pain Symptom Manage 1996;11(4):242–51.

45. Dillie KS, Fleming MF, Mundt MP, et al. Quality of life associated with daily opioid therapy in a primary care chronic pain sample. J Am Board Fam Med 2008;21(2):108–17.

46. Dawson R, Spross JA, Jablonski ES, et al. Probing the paradox of patients' satisfaction with inadequate pain management. J Pain Symptom Manage 2002;23(3): 211–20.
47. Ballantyne JC. Patient-centered health care: are opioids a special case? Spine J 2009;9:770–2.
48. McCracken LM, Klock PA, Mingay DJ, et al. Assessment of satisfaction with treatment for chronic pain. J Pain Symptom Manage 1997;14(5):292–9.
49. McNeill JA, Sherwood GD, Starck PL, et al. Assessing clinical outcomes: patient satisfaction with pain management. J Pain Symptom Manage 1998; 16(1):29–40.
50. Vila H, Smith RA, Augustyniak MJ, et al. The efficacy and safety of pain management before and after implementation of hospital-wide pain management standards: is patient safety compromised by treatment based solely on numerical pain ratings? Anesth Analg 2005;101:474–80.
51. Zacny J, Bigelow G, Compton P, et al. College on Problems of Drug Dependence Taskforce on prescription opioid non-medical use and abuse: position statement. Drug Alcohol Depend 2003;69(3):215–32.
52. AAPM Council on Ethics American Academy of Pain Medicine. Ethics Charter. 2005. Available at: http://www.painmed.org/productpub/pdfs/EthicsCharter.pdf. Accessed July 1, 2010.
53. Dubois MY. The birth of an ethics charter for pain medicine. Pain Med 2005;6(3): 201–2.
54. Joranson DE, Gilson AM. State intractable pain policy: current status. APS Bulletin 1997;7(2):7–9.
55. Grol R. Improving the quality of medical care: building bridges among professional pride, payer profit, and patient satisfaction. JAMA 2001;286(20):2578–85.
56. Aharony L, Strasser S. Patient satisfaction: what we know about and what we still need to explore. Med Care Rev 1993;50(1):49–79.
57. Heidegger T, Nuebling M, Saal D, et al. Patient-centered outcomes in clinical research: does it really matter? Br J Anaesth 2008;100(1):1–3.
58. Svensson I, Sjostrom B, Haljamae H. Influence of expectations and actual pain experiences on satisfaction with postoperative pain management. Eur J Pain 2001;5(2):125–33.
59. Thomas T, Robinson C, Champion D, et al. Prediction and assessment of the severity of post-operative pain and of satisfaction with management. Pain 1998;75(2–3):177–85.
60. Sullivan M. Ethical principles in pain management. Pain Med 2001;2:106–11.
61. Compton WM, Volkow ND. Major increases in opioid analgesic abuse in the United States: concerns and strategies. Drug Alcohol Depend 2006;81(2):103–7.
62. Paulozzi LJ, Budnitz DS, Xi Y. Increasing deaths from opioid analgesics in the United States. Pharmacoepidemiol Drug Saf 2006;15(9):618–27.
63. Kuehn BM. Opioid prescriptions soar: increase in legitimate use as well as abuse. JAMA 2007;17(3):249.
64. Eriksen J, Sjogren P, Bruera E, et al. Critical issues on opioids in chronic non-cancer pain. An epidemiological study. Pain 2006;125:172–9.
65. Wallace AS, Freburger JK, Darter JD, et al. Comfortably numb? Exploring satisfaction with chronic back pain visits. Spine J 2009;9(9):721–8.
66. Rubin SB. If we think it's futile, can't we just say no? HEC Forum 2007;19(1): 45–65.
67. Ballantyne JC, Fleisher LA. Ethical issues in opioid prescribing for chronic pain. Pain 2010;148(3):365–7.

Medication Safety in the Perioperative Setting

George M. Hanna, MD, Wilton C. Levine, MD*

KEYWORDS

• Medical errors • Medication errors • Perioperative safety

In 1999, the Institute of Medicine (IOM) reported that between 44,000 and 98,000 patients die annually as a result of preventable medical errors. These medical errors include adverse drug events, incorrect transfusion therapy, wrong-site surgery, and others. The IOM also found that at least 1.5 million preventable medication errors cause harm in the United States each year.[1] The IOM concluded that the most serious consequences of these errors occur in operating rooms, intensive care units, and emergency departments.[1]

Drug administration errors are a major cause of morbidity and mortality in hospitalized patients. These errors result in major harm and incur dramatic costs to the delivery of health care. In the United States, medication errors are estimated to cause approximately 7000 deaths per year.[2] Preventable drug errors are projected to directly cost a 700-bed teaching hospital $2.8 million annually,[3] based on postevent lengths of stay and total costs.

In health care, and especially in anesthesia, medication errors represent one of most prevalent contributors of iatrogenic injury.[4] The discipline of anesthesiology involves the delivery of multiple potent drugs, often given in rapid succession during high-acuity situations. The specialty is unique, as it is responsible for the direct preparation, dosing, and delivery of medications to patients by a physician and anesthesiologist, certified registered nurse anesthetist (CRNA), or anesthesia assistant (AA). In a survey of 687 Canadian anesthesiologists, 85% reported a drug error or near miss in clinical practice.[5] In a New Zealand study, 12.5% of practitioners surveyed reported that they were aware of causing harm to a patient because of a drug administration error.[4]

THE OPERATING ROOM MILIEU

The operating room is a distinct environment with a rapid workflow requiring immediate decisions and decision support. Research from the aviation industry indicates

Department of Anesthesia, Critical Care and Pain Medicine, 55 Fruit Street, Boston, MA 02114, USA
* Corresponding author.
E-mail address: Wlevine@partners.org

that errors occur more frequently in hectic, demanding and fast-paced environments,[6] such as the operating room. Best practice methods from elsewhere in the hospital, however, are not readily transferable and applicable to this setting. Despite persistent education and best efforts, errors continue to occur in the perioperative environment.

In most hospital areas, the typical workflow for medication administration to a patient involves important and time-consuming checks and balances (**Fig. 1**A). In this process, a physician first writes an order for a particular medication for a specific patient. A pharmacist then evaluates the order as it relates to the specific patient for appropriate dose, indication, patient allergy, and potential contraindications. The pharmacist next either approves the order or clarifies any questions. A nurse is next able to review the medication order in the hospital order entry system. If the

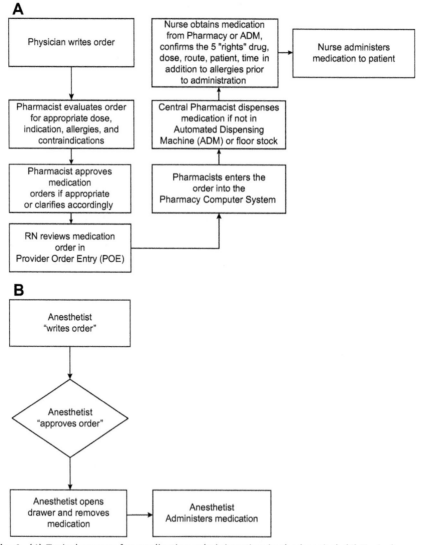

Fig. 1. (*A*) Typical process for medication administration in the hospital. (*B*) Typical process for medication administration in the operating room.

medication is stocked on the patient floor, the nurse may obtain access to the medication after this approval process; otherwise a pharmacist must dispense the medication to the patient location. Before administration of the medication to the patient, the nurse reviews the five medication rights: right patient, right time and frequency of administration, right dose, right route of administration and right drug. After completing all of these steps, the nurse administers the medication to the patient. Not surprisingly, this process can take hours to employ, with several checkpoints and hard stops before a subsequent step in the process is undertaken.

In the operating room, the process is dramatically abbreviated. The anesthetist internally writes an order, approves an order, prepares the medication, and administers the medication to a patient. This practice often takes seconds, and lacks the safeguards that exist in other areas of the hospital (see **Fig. 1**B).

TYPES OF MEDICATION ERRORS

Medication errors in anesthesia are not new, and unfortunately, they continue to occur despite being studied and reported since the earliest days of the specialty. Thirty years ago, Cooper and colleagues published a landmark study in anesthesia when they applied the model of critical incident reporting, a concept that originated in aviation, to the study of perioperative safety.[7,8] Critical incident analyses of major errors in anesthesia management revealed that human error was involved in nearly 70% of all events. One-fifth of all events discovered in this study were related to medication errors; yet of the incidents attributed to human error, approximately one-third were related to medications. Such events included inadvertent syringe substitutions, drug overdoses (syringe or vaporizer), and wrong choice of drugs. These findings began to bring awareness of patient safety to the fields of medicine and anesthesia.

A study by Webster and colleagues,[9] of nearly 8000 delivered anesthetics, reveals that one drug administration error occurs for every 133 anesthetics (0.75%) and a near-miss rate of 0.37% for all medication errors including boluses and infusions. The two largest categories of medication errors included incorrect dosing (20%) and accidental substitutions (20%). Sixty-three percent (63%) of all errors involved intravenous boluses. Amongs the intravenous bolus substitution errors, most occurred between different pharmacologic classes. These errors were implicated in subsequent negative outcomes, involving intraoperative awareness, prolonged mechanical ventilation, and transient physiologic effects requiring additional interventions. None of these reported errors resulted in death or permanent morbidity. More recent work, however, has approximated that 1 in every 250 drug errors is fatal.[10]

It is important to make a distinction between self-reporting studies and observational studies. The drug error rate of 0.75% as per Webster and colleagues may appear superior to error rates observed on medical wards (approximately 20%),[11] but it must be noted that voluntary reporting study designs are much less sensitive than observational studies.

Webster and colleagues[9] classify drug errors into the following categories

Omission—drug not given
Repetition—extra dose of an intended drug
Substitution—incorrect drug instead of the desired drug
Insertion—a drug that was not intended to be given at a particular time or at any time
Incorrect dose—wrong dose of an intended drug
Incorrect route—wrong route of an intended drug
Other—a complex event not falling into the previously mentioned categories.

Among 205 American Society of Anesthesiologists (ASA) closed claims for drug errors (representing 4% of all claims in the ASA Closed Claim Project Report in 2003), 31% of cases were described as incorrect dose; 24% were substitution, and 17% were cases of insertion. Other cases accounted for 24%.[12]

The similarity of medication names, drug vials, and label colors and frequently illegible documentation all play a major role in the occurrence of errors (**Fig. 2**). Additionally, the preparation of drugs and the need for specific calculations under time constraints may further promote medication errors. A medication error can be defined as an error in the prescription, dispensing, or administration of a drug with the result that the patient fails to receive the correct medication or the proper dosage.[13] In anesthesia, prescription refers to the decision of which drug to administer; dispensing refers to the selection of the drug from the pharmacy or anesthesia workstation along with the preparation of the drug, as medications are often transferred from vial to syringe, and administration describes the delivery of a drug to a patient.

In an effort to promote safe administration of medications to patients and to standardize labeling practice, the ASA has developed medication labeling standards, and The Joint Commission (TJC) has developed national patient safety goals promoting safe administration of medications. Drug labeling requires time and vigilance, is prone to human error, and is a major compliance issue when hospitals are being evaluated and accredited.[14,15] Incomplete labeling by clinicians is common (see **Fig. 2**A), along with medication labeling errors (see **Fig. 2**B). Medication labeling errors have been found to approach 10%. These incomplete and incorrect labels can lead to administration errors and faults in communication during handoffs and relief.[16]

While the ASA medication color labeling standards have been adopted by most anesthetists, practitioners have struggled to comply with TJC labeling standards, with less than 50% of syringe labels meeting TJC requirements.[14] This poor compliance causes one in five hospitals to be cited for poor medication labeling compliance on TJC surveys.[14] The preparation of medications and their appropriate labeling of medications by the anesthesiologist, CRNAs, or AAs, are brief processes that have potential pitfalls and barriers to accuracy and safety. TJC has specific requirements for labeling medications as a means of mitigating this problem. As a national patient safety goal, TJC instructs to "label all medications, medication containers (for example, syringes, medicine cups, basins), or other solutions on and off the sterile field."[15] Clinicians in the operating room understand the importance of drug labeling, but often find the time pressure too great to allow full compliance with the task. A 2004 study by the Institute of Safe Medication Practice (ISMP) found that 42% of clinicians label inconsistently.[16] For anesthetists in the operating room, there are many competing demands, ranging from the time required to fill out multiple fields to writing legibly on a small and sometimes wet label.

PERIOPERATIVE STANDARDS AND REGULATIONS

In January 2010, the Anesthesia Patient Safety Foundation (APSF) issued consensus recommendations on perioperative medication safety.[17] The APSF proposed a new paradigm built upon the traditional requirements of medication label formatting and an emphasis on the careful reading of labels. The APSF recommended a new paradigm of standardization, technology, pharmacy, and culture (SPTC).

Standardization

High alert drugs should be available in standardized concentrations/diluents prepared by pharmacy in a ready-to-use (bolus or infusion) form that is appropriate for both

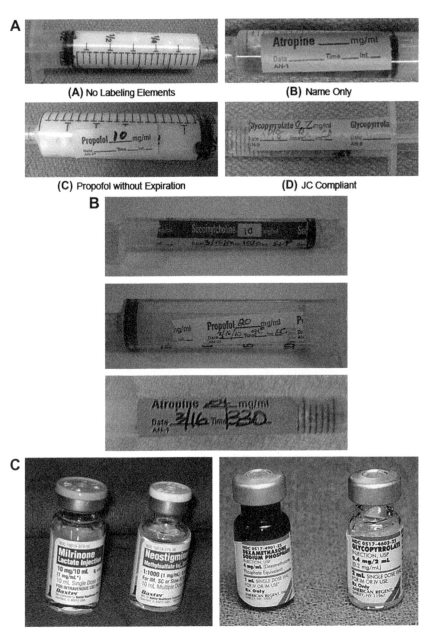

Fig. 2. (A) Medication labeling compliance in the operating room. (B) Medication labeling errors in the operating room—three different errors in drug concentration: Succinylcholine concentration listed as 10 mg/mL is actually 20 mg/mL; Propofol concentration listed as 20 mg/mL is actually 10 mg/mL; Atropine concentration listed as 0.04 mg/mL is actually 0.4 mg/mL. (C) Look-alike drug vials in the operating room.

adult and pediatric patients. Infusions should be delivered by an electronically controlled smart device containing a drug library. Ready-to-use syringes and infusions should have standardized fully compliant machine-readable labels.

Technology

Every anesthetizing location should have a mechanism to identify medications before drawing up or administering them (bar code reader) and a mechanism to provide feedback, decision support, and documentation (automated information system).

Pharmacy

Routine provider-prepared medications should be discontinued whenever possible. Clinical pharmacists should be part of the perioperative/operative room team. Standardized pre-prepared medication kits by case type should be used whenever possible.

Culture

Establish a just culture for reporting errors (including near misses) and discussion of lessons learned. Establish a culture of education, understanding, and accountability via a required curriculum and dissemination of dramatic stories. Establish a culture of cooperation and recognition of the benefits of these proposed changes within and between institutions, professional organizations, and accreditation agencies.

No matter how vigorously an individual or group of individuals attempts to perfect their drug delivery skills, human error persists. Health care professionals, who vow to protect patients from harm at all costs, must embrace this multifactorial approach to patient safety in the context of medication administration.

It is the duty of the anesthetist to care for and protect the patient during surgical procedures. It is crucial to understand the lapses in modern-day systems that lead to medication errors, so that they can be addressed and techniques optimized to keep patients from being harmed.

SOLUTIONS: TECHNIQUES AND TECHNOLOGY

Given the known potential harm and frequency of medication errors in the perioperative setting, several recommendations have been introduced in an effort to reduce these errors. Traditionally, providers have been encouraged to read labels carefully, up to three or four times for confirmation.[18] This simple technique may not suffice, as drug errors continue to occur in anesthesia and perioperative medicine.[5] An anesthesiologist administers over 500,000 drugs during a career,[5] and maintaining 100% accuracy is nearly impossible. Similar medication names, ambiguous or illegible labels on ampoules or syringes, and the lack of drug tray/cart standardization intertwined with intrinsic human factors continue to contribute to medication errors. The operating room environment, with abundant diversions and production pressures, dynamic physiologic changes in patients, and the potential for provider fatigue may all play key roles in errors.

Evidence-based solutions have been developed and studied to optimize the following objectives:

Compliance with regulatory standards and requirements
Elimination of medication delivery errors
Improvement in communication between providers
Improvement in real-time electronic documentation
Provide real-time clinical alerts.

Systematic review of the literature for recommendations that minimize errors in intravenous drug administration in anesthesia reveals strong suggestions[19]:

The label on any drug ampoule or syringe should be read carefully before a drug is drawn up or injected

The legibility and contents of labels on ampoules and syringes should be optimized according to agreed standards

Syringes should always be labeled

Formal organization of drug drawers and workspaces should be used

Labels should be checked with a second person or a device before a drug is drawn up or administered

Errors in intravenous drug administration during anesthesia should be reported and reviewed

Avoidance of similar packaging and presentation of drugs.

Modifications to the current system of practice to improve deficits in medication preparation, handling, and administration must be simple and easily integrated with operating room workflow. The implementation of standardization and technology to eliminate the human component has the potential of minimizing variability and inconsistency that leads to medication administration errors. Some of the solutions that have been developed and that are available will be discussed.

Many hospitals have begun using prefilled medication syringes. These syringes have the advantage of removing the necessary work of medication preparation and syringe labeling (transferring the medication from the vial to the syringe). Pharmacy compounding companies produce almost any medication and any concentration desired by clinicians. Individual anesthesia groups or hospitals can develop standard drug formularies, yet nationally there remains a struggle with consensus on a standardized drug formulary. This is also impacted currently by ongoing drug recalls.

Prefilled syringes are helpful for a portion of the anesthesiologist's work but do not completely address all of the practitioner's needs. Medications like propofol are not produced by compounding facilities. Other medications have only a 24-hour shelf life once transferred from the vial to the syringe or once they are diluted.

Some hospitals are developing in-house syringe preparation by using either pharmacy technicians or automated equipment such as the IntelliFill I.V. System (FHT, Inc, Daytona Beach, FL, USA). This system is designed to produce small-volume intravenous medications safely and quickly with a goal of improving medication safety.

In response to a report of 10,000 parenteral drug administration errors in the United Kingdom in 2006, 25 of which were fatal,[20] a technological solution, SAFERamp (Cambridge Enterprise, Ltd, Cambridge, UK), was developed. SAFERamp is a single-use ampoule opening and syringe-labeling device developed to increase safety and consistency while decreasing reliance on clinician accuracy in the preparation of medications. This process involves a syringe and ampoule apparatus that automatically labels the barrel of the syringe.

SAFERsleep is a system developed by Dr Merry's group in New Zealand. It is a system that uses bar-coded labels containing data for the drug name along with a standardized anesthesia drug tray. Upon administration, the clinician scans the medication's bar code containing medication name, and the system provides both a visual and auditory confirmation of the administration. The time of administration is recorded electronically, excluding the need for written documentation.

Other solutions have been developed in an attempt to improve patient safety and reduce the impact of human error during the delivery of drugs. Docusys provides a computerized interface for medication management, closed-loop narcotic tracking, and medication error prevention support through its optional pharmacy and point-of-care technology, integrating drug administration and automatic documentation of the medication and medication dose.

Safe Label System by Codonics, Incorporated, (Codonics Middleburg Heights, OH, USA) uses a bar code-assisted method of medication identification and labeling. The machine readily deciphers the US Food and Drug Administration (FDA)-required medication vial bar code, runs a series of safety checks on the drug vial, and then provides audio and visual confirmation of the medication name while printing a label. The printed label has information including drug name, concentration, date/time of preparation, date/time of expiration, user name/initials, and a barcode containing all this information that can be used at the time of medication administration to the patient. In clinical use, labeling compliance was found to be 100% with the Safe Label System compared with poor compliance rates with traditional/manual methods of labeling.[21] The time required to label medications with the Safe Label System was also faster compared with standard methods.[22]

Additional safety checks can be easily incorporated into new technological systems, without hindering workflow and convenience. Examination of medication recall and expiration, crosschecking for patient allergies, and real-time entry into the anesthesia record are all potential improvements that can keep patients safe during perioperative care. In addition, serialization of each bar code can allow safety checks that ensure syringes are not accidentally used on multiple patients.

REPORTING ERRORS: A NEW CULTURE

As the health care industry continues to be increasingly regulated, physicians must accept responsibility, assume transparency, and embrace accountability to maintain best practices for patients.

One can again learn from the aviation industry as a new culture that is a just culture and a nonpunitive setting are developed for reporting errors or near-miss events. In aviation, accidents and errors are treated as evidence of a damaged system. These events are perceived as prospective opportunities to remedy faults in an overall structural design. The Swiss cheese model of hazards leading to losses in the context of a chain of errors through successful layers of defenses and safeguards provides a system-based understanding of the causes of error (**Fig. 3**).[23]

In the operating room, multiple factors, including the prescriber, the drug administrator, the environment, the labels, and the formulations, all contribute to the medication delivery system and medication errors. Following an error, it may be easiest to blame an individual, but this is a culture that should be abandoned. An individualistic approach assigns blame and does not address the needed repair of broken systems. This rationale is unsound and often deters from the implementation of safety measures and honest reporting of lapses in an organizational schematic.

The development of modern reporting technologies in conjunction with quality assurance committees has led to potential improvements in transparency.[24] A nonputative forum is likely to promote the willingness of clinicians to account for errors and near misses. Physicians are not good reporters of errors, and this is exacerbated if there is a lack of objective feedback or presence of an impartial setting.[25] Opportunities to learn from errors require an integrated framework that is objective and can make formal recommendations on patient safety practices.[26] It has been shown that as more critical incidents are reported, the number of adverse events decreases.[27]

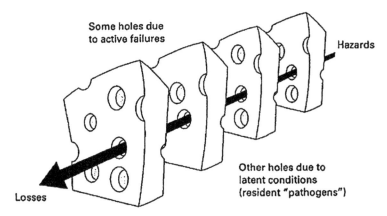

Fig. 3. The Swiss cheese model of accident causation. (*From* Reason J, Carthey J, deLeval M. Diagnosing "vulnerable system syndrome". An essential prerequisite to effective risk management. Qual Health Care 2001;10(Suppl II):ii21–5; with permission.)

SUMMARY

In an era of health care reform and increased emphasis on the elimination of preventable errors, physicians have a moral and legal imperative to adapt and improve patient safety practices. Modern-day society is unrelenting toward clinicians and hospitals committing clinical errors leading to serious consequences and injury to patients. In addition to the costs of human suffering, clinical errors have been implicated in the rising of health care expenditures. Medical errors lead to additional health care use, lost employment time and income, increased need for rehabilitation services, and disability, all estimated to cost between $17 billion and $29 billion annually.[1]

Medication errors in the perioperative setting have been studied and reviewed, and anesthesiologists have a crucial role in developing safe drug delivery strategies. The standardization of medications, in conjunction with the implementation of technological solutions to provide real-time feedback is necessary for optimizing patient safety. The promotion of a culture of accountability and increased transparency is needed to encourage clinicians to report errors, so that further analysis and recommendations can be provided. The process of reporting in a formal and unbiased forum helps a clinician understand the specific nature of the error, and an opportunity is given to rectify systems-based factors that may have contributed.

REFERENCES

1. Kohn LT, Corrigan JM, Donaldson MS. To err is human: building a safer health system. Committee on the Quality of Health Care in America, Institute of Medicine. Washington, DC: National Academy Press; 1999.
2. Phillips DP, Christenfeld N, Glynn LM. Increase in US medication error deaths between 1983 and 1993. Lancet 1998;351:643–4.
3. Bates DW, Spell N, Cullen DJ, et al. The costs of adverse drug events in hospitalized patients. Adverse Drug Events Prevention Study Group. J Am Med Assoc 1997;277:307–11.
4. Merry AF, Peck DJ. Anaesthetists, errors in drug administration, and the law. N Z Med J 1995;108:185–7.

5. Orser BA, Chen RJ, Yee DA. Medication errors in anesthetic practice: a survey of 687 practitioners. Can J Anaesth 2001;48:139–46.
6. Chou CD, Madhavian D, Funk K. Studies in cockpit task management errors. Int J Aviat Psychol 1996;6:307–20.
7. Cooper JB, Newbower RS, Long CD, et al. Preventable anesthesia mishaps—a study of human factors. Anesthesiology 1978;49:399–406.
8. Cooper JB, Newbower RS, Kitz RJ. An analysis of major errors and equipment failures in anesthesia management: considerations for prevention and detection. Anesthesiology 1984;60:34–42.
9. Webster CS, Merry AF, Larsson L, et al. The frequency and nature of drug administration error during anaesthesia. Anaesth Intensive Care 2001;29:494–500.
10. Stabile M, Webster CS, Merry AF. Medication administration in anesthesia: time for a paradigm shift. APSF Newsletter 2007;22:44–6.
11. Barker KN, Flynn EA, Pepper GA, et al. Medication errors observed in 36 health care facilities. Arch Intern Med 2002;162:1897–903.
12. Bowdle TA. Drug administration errors from the ASA closed claims project. ASA Newsl 2003;67:11–3.
13. Wheeler SJ, Wheeler DW. Medication errors in anaesthesia and critical care. Anaesthesia 2005;60:257–73.
14. Top standard compliance issues for first half 2007. Jt Comm Perspect 2008;28:1–3.
15. Suyderhoud JP. Joint Commission on Accreditation of Healthcare Organizations requirements and syringe labeling systems. Anesth Analg 2007;104:242.
16. Institute for Safe Medication Practices (ISMP) medication safety self-assessment. Available at: http://www.ismp.org. Accessed December 22, 2010.
17. Eichhorn JH. APSF hosts medication safety conference: consensus group defines challenges and opportunities for improved practice. APSF Newsletter 2010;25:1–20.
18. Mangar D, Miguel R, Villarreal JR. Reporting every look alike is no longer novel: similarities between labels are a fact of life. J Clin Anesth 1992;4:347–8.
19. Jensen LS, Merry AF, Webster CS, et al. Evidence-based strategies for preventing drug administration errors during anaesthesia. Anaesthesia 2004;59:493–504.
20. Promoting safer use of injectable medicines. London (UK): British NHS/National Patient Safety Agency; 2007.
21. Vernest KA, Nanji (Caputo) K, Driscoll WD, et al. Smart labels: improving syringe labeling compliance and patient safety in the operating room. Presented at the ASA Conference, 2009. New Orleans (LA). October 17–21, 2009.
22. Caputo (Nanji) K, Vernest KA, Driscoll WD, et al. Smart labels: improving syringe labeling efficiency and accuracy in the operating room. Presented at the ASA Conference, 2009. New Orleans (LA). October 17–21, 2009.
23. Reason J. Human error: models and management. BMJ 2000;320:768–70.
24. Mahajan RP. Critical incident reporting and learning. Br J Anaesth 2010;105:69–75.
25. Sanghera IS, Franklin BD, Dhillon S. The attitudes and beliefs of healthcare professionals on the causes and reporting of medication errors in a UK intensive care unit. Anaesthesia 2007;62:53–61.
26. Runciman WB, Williamson JAH, Deakin A, et al. An integrated framework for safety quality and risk management: an information and incident management system based on a universal patient safety classification. Qual Saf Health Care 2006;15:i82–90.
27. National Patient Safety Agency. Seven steps to patient safety: an overview guide for NHS staff. Available at: http://www.nrls.npsa.nhs.uk/resources. Accessed December 22, 2010.

Reduction of Regulated Medical Waste Using Lean Sigma Results in Financial Gains for Hospital

Jerry Stonemetz, MD[a],*, Julius C. Pham, MD, PhD[b],
Alejandro J. Necochea, MD, MPH[c], John McGready, PhD, MS[d],
Robert E. Hody, BSEE, MSEE, MSCS, CMBB[e],
Elizabeth A. Martinez, MD, MHS[f]

KEYWORDS

• Medical waste • Reduction • Lean Sigma • Financial gains

Hospitals in the United States are facing increased financial pressures, and many are focused on waste reduction efforts. By 2007, the annual cost of health care in the United States was greater than 2.2 trillion dollars.[1] With the depressed economy, struggling US hospitals are keeping aged equipment, reducing staff, and changing purchasing practices to cut costs. However, these cuts may increase staff workloads and stress and may directly or indirectly decrease the safety of patients.[2]

Partial salary support was provided to Dr Stonemetz for this effort during a fellowship program with the Center of Innovations in Quality Patient Care at the Johns Hopkins University.
There are no conflicts of interest to acknowledge.
[a] Department Anesthesia & Critical Care Medicine, Johns Hopkins University, Baltimore, MD, USA
[b] Departments of Emergency Medicine, and Anesthesia and Critical Care Medicine, Quality and Safety Research Group, Johns Hopkins University, School of Medicine, 1909 Thames Avenue, Baltimore, MD 21231, USA
[c] Department of Internal Medicine, Johns Hopkins School of Medicine, 5200 Eastern Avenue, MFL Building West Tower 6F, Baltimore, MD 21224, USA
[d] Department of Biostatistics, Johns Hopkins Bloomberg School of Public Health, 615 North Wolfe Street, Baltimore, MD 21205, USA
[e] Center for Innovation in Quality Patient Care, 601 North Caroline Street, Baltimore, MD 21287, USA
[f] Department of Anesthesia, Critical Care and Pain Medicine, Massachusetts General Hospital, Harvard University, 55 Fruit Street, Boston, MA 02114, USA
* Corresponding author.
E-mail address: Jstonemetz@jhmi.edu

Anesthesiology Clin 29 (2011) 145–152
doi:10.1016/j.anclin.2010.11.007
1932-2275/11/$ – see front matter

Process improvement in health care typically involves efforts to improve patient outcomes or increase patient safety; however, there is a significant need to make health care more cost-effective, in part from reduction of unnecessary waste, such as in costs or use of resources. Using a manufacturing methodology called Lean Six Sigma, many health care facilities are beginning to attempt to reduce waste and improve care by using the lean component to reduce waste, and then the Six Sigma methodology to reduce variation in processes.[3] In the lexicon of lean methodologies, identifying muda (waste that can be eliminated without affecting outcomes) has become the cornerstone of reducing unnecessary steps, expenses, and wasteful processes.[4] There are examples in the literature that highlight experiences that are focused on reducing waste. Examples from the anesthesia literature include efforts to reduce the waste of medication use in the delivery of an anesthetic and in the elimination of unnecessary preoperative testing.[5–9]

Weinger[9] discussed the use of appropriate anesthetic agents and the wasting of drugs that have been procured but never used during an anesthetic as it relates to the routine cost of care for an anesthetic, and Smith[8] described considerations when targeting anesthetic drug waste reduction efforts. Another area of interest has been the elimination of unnecessary preoperative testing. Roizen[6] has long argued that there are substantial savings possible with more focused testing, and advocates of preoperative algorithms and protocols show that these mechanisms can help to reduce unnecessary testing, but they are rarely used to any great extent.[5]

There is a broad range of other opportunities within the health care environment to reduce costs and waste that would not jeopardize the safety of patients or providers. One area is regulated medical waste (RMW) disposal. Although there are few scientific articles defining the precise amount of medical waste (trash), there is consensus among all stakeholders that there is substantial inappropriate excess that could, and should, be eliminated. The Occupational Safety and Health Administration (OSHA) defines regulated waste as any trash that contains bodily fluid in an amount that may splatter when compressed or is saturated enough to cake and contaminate on transfer (US Department of Labor, OSHA. Regulations (Standards 29CFR) Bloodborne pathogens. http://www.osha.gov/pls/oshaweb/owadisp.show_document?p_table=STANDARDS&p_id=10051 [accessed March 21, 2010]). RMW costs more to process than regular waste. After multiple incidents of needles washing up on beaches, OSHA passed the Medical Waste Tracking Act of 1988 and began regulating hospital waste. Hospitals typically ship RMW to intermediaries who process this regulated waste at a cost of 6 to 10 times more than conventional waste disposal. At our institution, it costs 24.5 cents/lb to dispose of RMW compared with 4 center per pound (lb) for regular waste, where 1 lb = 0.45 kilograms, resulting in a cost differential of 20.5 cents/lb for RMW. This cost differential is similar to that of other institutions. We hypothesized that conventional waste was being added to red bags and increasing the volume of RMW.

This study assesses the waste disposal process in the surgical suites of an academic medical center and uses a process improvement methodology to decrease the volume and costs of RMW.

METHODS

This was a prospective study of RMW in the surgical suites of a large urban academic medical center from January 2007 to December 2008. Adult, pediatric, and outpatient (attached surgicenter) suites were included. The combined average annual surgical volume for the institution is more than 40,000 cases. We used a methodology called Lean Six Sigma, which uses the lean approach of reducing waste and inefficiencies, and then implements Six Sigma methodology to reduce variation in the process.[3] Lean principles guide the process of analyzing every step and every supply in every process to identify steps or supplies in the process that are nonessential and can potentially be eliminated. Six Sigma uses specific statistical principles to guide the identification and reduction of variation in processes.

Initially, a charter team was formed for the Lean Six Sigma process. This team was championed and led by an anesthesiologist (JS) trained in Lean Six Sigma methodology and was composed of hospital administrators, operating room (OR) personnel and managers, and internal Lean Six Sigma experts (RH). The Lean Six Sigma methodology uses 5 steps: define, measure, analyze, improve, and control (DMAIC) (**Fig. 1**).[10] We systematically applied these steps to study and improve the RMW disposal process.

To define the problem, the charter team reviewed hospital-wide RMW volume and cost of disposal as reported directly from Environmental Services' budgets. At baseline, this institution produced 15 million pounds of trash per year at an annual cost in excess of US$3 million. The RMW represented 47.24% of the total waste stream, which is notably higher than the reported national average of 15%.[11] The charter team spent 2 days visually inspecting waste collected in red trash bags throughout the surgical suites, and determined that much of the waste contents were not appropriate for RMW disposal, as defined by OSHA. Therefore, reducing the amount of RMW was identified as a concrete problem with a measurable outcome.

To measure and analyze the problem, we targeted ORs where a large portion of the hospital's hazardous waste is produced. We measured RMW in pounds per month and total waste in pounds per month. Analysis of cost savings was accomplished by multiplying the RMW by a cost differential of 20.5 cents/lb (differential calculated

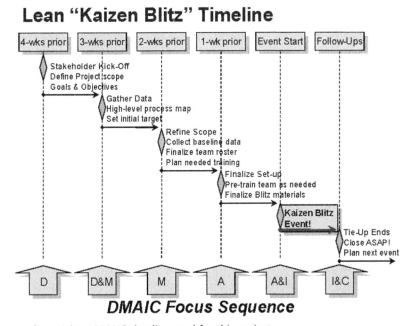

Fig. 1. A lean Kaizen DMAIC timeline used for this project.

as 24.5 cents/lb for RMW minus 4 cents/lb for municipal trash), and then subtracting this from the total cost of all hospital waste during fiscal year 2007.

To develop improvement strategies, the charter team identified stakeholders directly involved in the RMW disposal process. Nurses *in* operating rooms and *postanesthesia care units* (PACU), OR technicians, anesthesiologists, and Environmental Services personnel were included. The team also identified individuals with regulatory or administrative jurisdiction over the process (eg, safety officers, nurse educators, and hospital administrative staff) and invited them to join the improvement team. These stakeholders attended a 1-day Kaizen Blitz event on January 11, 2007, which is a rapid improvement method used in Lean Sigma. The Blitz event typically requires a detailed mapping of the process, the identification of issues or obstacles needing improvement, and improvement requirements that must be met.

For the control step, the improvement team developed an action plan to reduce the volume of RMW generated in one of the hospital's OR/PACU areas. The action plan was pilot tested in the primary OR/PACU area for 4 weeks, and subsequently extended to the other operating locations in the hospital (40 additional ORs).

IMPLEMENTATION OF IMPROVEMENT PLAN

Strategies defined by the improvement team included (1) clarification of the guidelines for what constitutes RMW versus municipal trash as defined by OSHA, (2) identification of procedure areas needing additional receptacles of each kind, (3) designing and posting clear signage for receptacles and educational posters, and (4) developing an education plan for all staff. The improvement plan was implemented within 1 week of defining improvement strategies in the pilot OR/PACU area and piloted for an additional 3 weeks. The improvement plan was then extended to the remainder of general operating room suites of the hospital beginning in April 2007.

STATISTICAL ANALYSIS

Descriptive statistics (means and proportions) were used to describe municipal waste, RMW, total medical waste (TMW), and RMW as a proportion of TMW. The cost of RMW management was calculated based on the following formula: cost of RMW (\$) = RMW (lb)×0.245 (\$). Differences in the weight of medical waste were compared using the *t*-test with unequal variances. A linear regression was performed to assess the effect of the intervention on TMW, RMW, and RMW as a proportion of TMW as a function of time. A linear spline was created at the start of the intervention. Potential savings were calculated by subtracting the average cost of RMW management during the baseline period from the cost of RMW management during the study period, and extrapolating this for the 24-month study period. A 2-way P value of .05 or less was considered statistically significant in all analyses. Analyses were performed using STATA 8.2 (College Station, TX, USA).

RESULTS

Observation of the waste disposal process in the OR/PACU revealed separate containers for RMW and municipal waste (clear bags). However, clear bags were frequently missing, mislabeled, or of poor quality, leading to disposal of regular garbage in RMW containers. Visual inspection of the contents of RMW containers revealed that approximately 80% was not RMW, as defined by OSHA, and should have been disposed of as municipal waste.

During the study period, the change in total waste was not statistically significant (1.3 million lb in January 2007, 1.1 million lb in December 2008, mean 1241,561 ± 79,861 lb /mo, P = .39). The amount of RMW as a percentage of total hospital waste decreased from 50% at baseline to 38% at the 24-month postintervention period, a decline of 12% (**Fig. 2**). As a proportion of the total waste, the RMW declined throughout the study period by approximately 0.55% (95% confidence interval [CI] 0.43–0.67) per month.

There was a 30% reduction in RMW per month from baseline (618,130 lb) to the last month of the study (432,367 lb). Before intervention, the RMW was stable (see **Fig. 2**). Throughout the study period, there was an approximate 7821 lb (95% CI 6190–9452) decline of RMW per month compared with the baseline period (see **Fig. 2**). Overall, the average RMW in the baseline period was 618,130 ± 17,122 lb per month compared with 520,167 ± 13,093 lb per month during the study period, showing a difference of 97,964 lb (95% CI 51,681–144,246) per month.

The cost of RMW declined throughout the study period by approximately $1916 (95% CI 1516–2316) per month compared with the baseline period. Overall, the average cost of RMW management in the baseline period was $151,442 ± 4195 per month compared with $127,441 ± 3208 per month in the study period, saving $24,001 (95% CI 12,662–35,340) per month on RMW disposal. At baseline it cost $151,442 per month for RMW disposal compared with $105,930 for the last month of the study period, leading to a $45,512/mo decline in the cost of RMW management. The potential saving in RMW was $576,024 for the institution.

DISCUSSION

This project reduced the volume of RMW in the main surgical suites of a large urban academic medical center and saved the institution $576,024 in the 24-month period. This paper shows the successful implementation of Lean Six Sigma methodology in the reduction of RMW in a large tertiary care center. Although there have been other studies of trash reduction in health care settings,[11,12] this paper is a unique example of how the anesthesiologist can play an important leadership role in the design and management of process improvement projects focused on reducing waste.

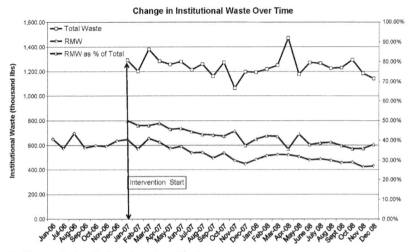

Fig. 2. Change in institutional waste with time.

In today's health care environment, many hospitals are struggling to maintain profitability. As a result, tough decisions are being made regarding operational expenses that may harm patients and affect employees. Hospital leaders looking for opportunities to lower expenses should turn to those at the frontline who can identify waste (eg, unnecessary costs or steps in a process) in the delivery of care. There have been estimates that hospitals produce 4 billion tons of trash per year, of which approximately 15% to 20% is RMW.[11,13] This represents a significant national cost that could be reduced substantially if RMW was reduced to less than 5% of the trash stream; a goal that has been established by the Hospitals for a Healthy Environment coalition (Practice Greenhealth. Reducing regulated medical waste. http://cms.h2e-online.org/ee/rmw/reducermw/).

We showed that anesthesiologists are in the position to take a leadership role in the design and management of a process improvement project that reduced unnecessary waste. Many anesthesiologists focus their quality improvement efforts on processes pertaining to patient care; however, some also see hospital RMW reduction by anesthesia as an important area that can tie process improvement to direct savings for the institution.[14] We encourage anesthesiologists to expand process improvement efforts to areas beyond patient care and those that may have an effect on the financial success of our facilities.

Successful approaches to RMW reduction have been described,[15,16] including an abstract using the plan-do-study-act cycle for continuous improvement.[16] However, this is the first paper that focuses on using Lean Six Sigma in the operating room to reduce RMW. The Lean Sigma strategies emphasize the use of multidisciplinary teams to identify the problems and the solutions. The proposed interventions in this initiative included staff education, clarification of policies, renegotiation of waste management contracts, as well as improvement of containers and implements used to dispose of RMW.

We have shown a significant and sustainable reduction of RMW production through the systematic use of the Lean Sigma methodology. There are important advantages to using the Lean Six Sigma approach, with a Kaizen event, for such efforts. First, the improvement team in this project was able to quickly identify the problem. We developed and implemented a strategy that produced results within weeks and could sustain these results.

Second, Lean Six Sigma emphasizes that solutions are generated by the frontline users who work in the process. The sense of group ownership of the process and the empowerment of individual participants inherent in the Lean Sigma methodology help make the solutions sustainable. In organizations with the ability to adapt quickly and with committed stakeholders, strategies for improvement can be developed and implemented rapidly. Although the Kaizen event was convened to address the RMW problem in a particular OR/PACU area in the hospital, many of the stakeholders involved had jurisdiction over the process throughout the hospital, which helped disseminate the intervention to other areas. We believe that the dramatic decrease in RMW volumes seen throughout 2007 (see **Fig. 2**) and sustained through 2008 represents the adoption and spread of the improvement strategies throughout the institution.

It is imperative that physicians, nursing staff, and other clinical, administrative, and environmental service staff are all engaged for this type of project. It requires a strong clinical champion and comprehensive management participation to bring about this type of change, despite being an obvious cost reduction, good for the environment, and simply the right thing to do. Successful implementation of this level of waste segregation requires a grassroots commitment to reducing RMW.

There are several potential limitations to this study. First, these results may have been due to the Hawthorne effect; that is, personnel were reducing RMW because they were being studied. However, the sustained and continued reduction in RMW suggests that the results persisted long after the Kaizen event. Second, the baseline period was short. Third, our cost savings projections did not include the cost of the project (eg, staff time, implementation of strategies). We did not keep a record of individual hours contributed to this project. All effort was contributed within the employees' standard work duties. Therefore, these cost estimates are slightly overestimated. Fourth, our percentage of RMW was much higher than the national average, and it may not be possible to generalize this approach to cost reduction to institutions that have a much lower percentage of RMW. The high percentage of RMW may be secondary to our facility being an academic institution; nonetheless, it illustrates that, although we have made progress to date, there is still opportunity for improvement. Nevertheless, we have shown that, in our institution, this proved to be an effective cost-reduction strategy and we would advocate that institutions evaluate their current practices. We did not intend to compare Lean Six Sigma methodology with other leadership paradigms so cannot make a conclusion that this approach is better than other quality improvement designs (eg, plan-do-study-act) or different leadership types (eg, nursing or environment services). However, we argue that this type of cross-discipline quality improvement work is well suited to having an anesthesiologist lead.

In conclusion, we advocate that anesthesiologists become familiar with Lean Six Sigma in an effort to make process improvement a more robust effort at their institutions. Developing important partnerships with hospitals and hospital leaders and aligning financial incentives can create a stronger position, especially as financial pressures become greater. In addition to facilitating better financial strength, it is important for all of us to be aware of our ability to affect our carbon footprint and strive to emulate many other industries in reducing our effect on our environment.

ACKNOWLEDGMENTS

The authors would like to acknowledge Christine G. Holzmueller, BLA, for her assistance in editing this manuscript and Chris Seale, director of Environmental Services for his assistance in procuring data for this project.

REFERENCES

1. Hartman M, Martin A, McDonnell P, et al. National health spending in 2007: slower drug spending contributes to lowest rate of overall growth since 1998. Health Aff (Millwood) 2009;28:246–61.
2. Kane RL, Shamliyan T, Mueller C, et al. Nurse staffing and quality of patient care. Evid Rep Technol Assess (Full Rep) 2007;151:1–115.
3. George M, Rowlands D, Kastle B. What is Lean Sigma? New York: McGraw-Hill; 2004.
4. Varkey P, Reller MK, Resar RK. Basics of quality improvement in health care. Mayo Clin Proc 2007;82:735–9.
5. Garcia-Miguel FJ, Serrano-Aguilar PG, Lopez-Bastida J. Preoperative assessment. Lancet 2003;362:1749–57.
6. Roizen MF. Preoperative evaluation of patients: a review. Ann Acad Med Singapore 1994;23:49–55.
7. Roizen MF. Cost-effective preoperative laboratory testing. JAMA 1994;271: 319–20.

An Anesthesiology Department Leads Culture Change at a Hospital System Level to Improve Quality and Patient Safety

Peter M. Fleischut, MD[a,d],*, Adam S. Evans, MD, MBA[b,d], Susan L. Faggiani, RN, BA, CPHQ[c,d], Eliot J. Lazar, MD, MBA[d,e,f], Gregory E. Kerr, MD, MBA[d,g,h]

KEYWORDS

- Housestaff quality council • Culture change
- Quality and patient safety • Quality improvement

When one does a Google search for "housestaff culture," one is referred to many sites dealing with the culture of the White House staff and even more on how residents should obtain, handle, and evaluate bacterial cultures. According to the Accreditation Council on Graduate Medical Education (ACGME), medical housestaff—residents and

The authors have no financial disclosures or conflicts of interests.

[a] Department of Anesthesiology, New York-Presbyterian Hospital, Weill Cornell Medical College, 525 East 68th Street, M-308, Box 124, New York, NY 10065, USA

[b] Department of Anesthesiology, New York-Presbyterian Hospital, Columbia Presbyterian Medical Center, 630 West 168th Street, New York, NY 10032, USA

[c] Department of Anesthesiology, New York-Presbyterian Hospital, Weill Cornell Medical College, 525 East 68th Street, A-1014, Box 124, New York, NY 10065, USA

[d] Housestaff Quality Council, New York-Presbyterian Hospital, 525 East 68th Street, M-308, Box 124, New York, NY 10065, USA

[e] Department of Medicine, New York-Presbyterian Hospital, Weill Cornell Medical College, 525 East 68th Street, New York, NY 10065, USA

[f] Department of Public Health, New York-Presbyterian Hospital, Weill Cornell Medical College, 525 East 68th Street, New York, NY 10065, USA

[g] Department of Anesthesiology, New York-Presbyterian Hospital, Weill Cornell Medical College, 525 East 68th Street, Box 124, New York, NY 10065, USA

[h] Critical Care Services, New York-Presbyterian Hospital, 525 East 68th Street, New York, NY 10065, USA

* Corresponding author. Department of Anesthesiology, New York-Presbyterian Hospital, Weill Cornell Medical College, 525 East 68th Street, M-308, Box 124, New York, NY 10065.
E-mail address: pmf9003@med.cornell.edu

fellows—make up one-seventh of all active physicians in the United States at any given point in time.[1] Despite their central role in the health workforce, few people have looked at the cultural changes associated with these postgraduate trainees who are intimately involved and embedded in our nation's health care system. Yet one cannot overestimate the importance of the culture of physician housestaff (residents and fellows) and the impact that it has on the delivery of patient care. The fact that there are 109,000 residents and fellows out of a total of slightly more than 700,000 physicians in the United States demonstrates the significant role of the housestaff.[1,2] Thus, the residents' knowledge base, clinical skills, attitudes, goals, and behavior, ie, the housestaff culture, greatly affect our nation's health care order.

The past decade has seen the emergence of the Joint Commission National Patient Safety Goals, the Centers for Medicare and Medicaid Services (CMS) Quality Program, the Leapfrog Group, Reasonably Preventable Conditions, and various quality initiatives such as the 2004 Institute for Healthcare Improvement's 100,000 Lives campaign to avoid unnecessary deaths (deaths deemed to be avoidable in hospital settings). When one attends seminars or conferences dealing with the issues, it is rare to see housestaff present to become involved in discussions around the best way to address these goals or to communicate the message. Given that residents provide a significant percentage of patient care at academic institutions, their involvement would seem to be of great importance. It appears that another cultural transformation is in order.

It is unusual for hospitals with residency programs to have formal systems in place where ongoing communication between key stakeholders in the hospital work regularly with housestaff to generate policies and procedures that have the goals of optimizing patient care and safety. Members of the Department of Anesthesiology at New York-Presbyterian Hospital, Weill Cornell Medical Center recognized this shortcoming and the need for culture change by proposing a systematic approach to involvement of housestaff in quality and patient safety (QPS) matters in a more meaningful way.

The chair of the Department of Anesthesiology at New York-Presbyterian Hospital (NYP), Weill Cornell Medical Center has supported and actively encouraged members of the department to pursue their particular interests. Indeed, leadership like this fosters creativity, ingenuity, and productivity. Because of this, many members of the faculty and staff in the department are intimately involved in the affairs of the hospital. Many, either directly or indirectly, oversee clinical care of patients in the operating rooms, the postoperative anesthesia care units, the pain management clinic, and some of the intensive care units. Many of them chair some of the most influential clinical committees in the hospital.

Over the years, it became clear to many of the faculty and staff that a key partner in patient care, the resident, was rarely present at clinical committee meetings with the ability to give input on important issues. As members of the department tried to understand how best to engage the housestaff into quality improvement efforts, it became clear that housestaff had to be equally involved in the planning process. There was a strong belief that an environment where housestaff felt empowered would result in a culture where housestaff would be motivated to deliver optimal patient care. It was felt that this cultural transformation could be accomplished by engaging housestaff in the generation of policies and decisions that involved patient care and safety, thereby empowering residents to provide the best patient care possible.

In 2008, members of the Department of Anesthesiology at New York-Presbyterian Hospital, Weill Cornell Medical College presented the concept of a GME-focused effort in quality and patient safety. The centerpiece for this initiative and the highlight of the vision was the creation of the Housestaff Quality Council (HQC). The HQC is composed of resident representatives of all the clinical departments in the institution who assumed the role of facilitators of the culture change.

There have been huge cultural shifts with regard to the housestaff experience over the past 50 years. In the 1970s, housestaff activism compelled hospitals to improve working conditions as well as improve compensation. In the 1980s, housestaff in New York State started to work shorter hours owing to legislation passed by the New York State legislature. In 2003, the Patient and Physician Safety Act was passed by Congress to address patient safety and resident work hours, as well as sleep deprivation. Not only do housestaff get paid more and work fewer hours, they now feel empowered to ensure that the work hour regulations get enforced. Improved patient care delivery will be the result of empowering the housestaff in ways that incite them to enhance the care they deliver.

CREATION OF THE HOUSESTAFF QUALITY COUNCIL BY THE DEPARTMENT OF ANESTHESIOLOGY
Hospital Background

NYP is the largest hospital in New York and one of the most comprehensive university hospitals in the country, with leading specialists in every field of medicine. It is one medical center with several campuses, affiliated with 2 highly regarded, Ivy League medical schools: Weill Cornell Medical College of Cornell University and Columbia University College of Physicians and Surgeons.

This 2298-bed hospital provides state-of-the-art inpatient, ambulatory, and preventive care in all areas of medicine. The hospital includes several facilities: NYP-Weill Cornell Center, NYP-Columbia Presbyterian Center, The Allen Hospital, Morgan Stanley Children's Hospital of New York-Presbyterian, and NYP Hospital/Westchester Division.

Preliminary Discussions

In 2008, the medical director of the Cardiothoracic Intensive Care Unit (CT-ICU), an anesthesiologist, approached two CA-1 residents in anesthesiology to discuss the creation of a quality improvement project in the CT-ICU. The residents had a particular interest in QPS matters stemming from medical school days and were eager to make a contribution. While discussing this project and its potential merits, it became apparent to the CT-ICU medical director that housestaff in anesthesiology, as well as other clinical departments, had minimal input in strategic planning or daily operations at the hospital when adverse events occurred or problems were identified. They were caring for patients in their own silos, generally not engaged in QPS issues, either at the hospital or departmental level. Simultaneously, it was noted that at hospital operational meetings and conferences, the "preachers were preaching to the choir," ie, hospital leadership was addressing issues to those already aware of them whereas those who were not aware, the housestaff, were not present to participate in these discussions. The housestaff as front-line caregivers were not at the table participating in these discussions about QPS and for any change to occur, a drastic cultural shakeup was needed.[3,4]

This preliminary discussion quickly shifted to the need for housestaff involvement in QPS matters and policy decision making, with an alteration in the traditional role of the housestaff in their relationship with hospital leadership. As a result, the CT-ICU medical director suggested that the residents explore the development of a group to engage residents in the hospital's quality and patient safety activities.[3,4]

To frame this project, the residents approached the QPS administrator in the Department of Anesthesiology to learn about some of the current QPS projects and concerns in the department. Early on, they determined that some of the departmental concerns were likely similar to those in other clinical departments. Speaking with resident colleagues in other departments, the residents in anesthesiology thought that there was enough interest to proceed with conducting a research study aimed at improving patient care and safety by promoting housestaff participation in policy and decision making. With the urging of the CT-ICU medical director, and from these preliminary discussions, the HQC was born.

Presentation to Senior Hospital Leadership

To begin the process of creating the HQC, the residents needed buy-in and approval from senior leadership at the hospital. They needed to convince senior leadership that if their ideas could be heard in a formalized manner, the housestaff could play a key role in making improvements in the daily operations of the hospital. If the culture at the hospital was to change, formal 2-way communication needed to be established.[3]

Working with the CT-ICU medical director and the departmental QPS administrator, the residents developed a presentation and invited the chief medical officer, the vice president of medical affairs/designated institutional official, the chief QPS officer, and vice presidents of quality and patient safety to meet with them. The presentation focused on several components:

- *The Current Milieu*: As key partners in patient care, and frequently involved in sentinel events, the housestaff were not routinely included in discussions and decision making regarding policy changes, inadvertently creating an "us" versus "them" environment. In an environment of public reporting, it seemed essential to involve housestaff in moving the needle to improved processes and outcomes.
- *The Mission*: To improve patient care and patient safety at NYP by creating a culture that promotes greater housestaff participation.
- The Proposal:
  1. "Buy-in" through involvement in policy making
  2. Dissemination of knowledge to peers
  3. Enforcement of best practices and policies
  4. Development of relationships
  5. Communication of key changes
  6. Measurement of how we are doing.

The presentation was received enthusiastically and the senior leadership group endorsed the proposal.[4]

Tracking the Change in Culture

Cultural change is difficult to assess. How do you evaluate the effect of what you have done and whether your actions have resulted in a major influence on an organization's culture? In an environment where the hospital was continually initiating changes to improve quality and patient safety, how could the introduction of the HQC and their involvement in quality and patient safety be assessed?

As the members of the Department of Anesthesiology started the HQC, the founding members wanted to establish a baseline of housestaff attitude and assess the culture toward quality and patient safety. Partnering with Dr Bryan Sexton, formerly of Johns Hopkins University and currently at Duke University, an attitudinal survey was used to assess housestaff attitude and culture. In the past, this survey had been distributed throughout the country to assess hospital-based culture.

Institutional review board approval was obtained and the survey was distributed to the entire housestaff in September 2008. Since the initial distribution, the survey has been repeated in 9-month intervals over the past 3 years, and has been slightly modified to include measurement of interdepartmental communication. The most recent version of the survey is shown in **Fig. 1**.

The initial survey showed that the housestaff were neutral in their view of QPS and demonstrated that they were not engaged in QPS at the hospital, as seen in the sample of survey questions shown in **Table 1**.[5]

These data suggested that improvement could be made in quality and patient safety by engaging housestaff in the policy and decision-making processes of the hospital.

IRB Protocol #0807009889
New York Presbyterian Hospital-Weill Cornell Medical College Safety Attitudes Survey

My participation in this minimal-risk survey study is entirely voluntary. During the course of this study, the research team of the Weill Cornell Medical College (WCMC) will be collecting information that they may share with New York Presbyterian Hospital-Weill Cornell Medical College administration, study monitors who check the accuracy of the information, and individuals who put all the study information together in report form. No identifying information will be collected. I understand that I may refuse to answer any (or all) of the questions at this or any other time. By answering the questions, I am providing authorization for the research team to use and share this information at any time. If I do not want to authorize the use and disclosure of this information, I may choose not to answer these questions and my status and the relationship with WCMC will not be affected by it. There is no expiration date for the use of this information as stated in this authorization. This process will be repeated every eight months until August of 2011.

Department: _____   Training Level: PGY-___   Gender: Male / Female

Did you complete this survey in 2009? Yes / No / Don't Know

Are you a member of the Housestaff Quality Council? Yes / No / Don't Know

Please choose your responses using the scale below:

1	2	3	4	5	X
Disagree Strongly	Disagree Slightly	Neutral	Agree Slightly	Agree Strongly	Not Applicable

1.	It is difficult to speak up if I perceive a problem with patient care.	1	2	3	4	5	X
2.	I have the support I need from other personnel to care for patients.	1	2	3	4	5	X
3.	It is easy for personnel here to ask questions when there is something that they do not understand.	1	2	3	4	5	X
4.	The physicians and nurses here work together as a well-coordinated team.	1	2	3	4	5	X
5.	I would feel safe being treated here as a patient.	1	2	3	4	5	X
6.	The Housestaff Quality Council has improved patient safety	1	2	3	4	5	X
7.	I know the proper channels to direct questions regarding patient safety in the hospital.	1	2	3	4	5	X
8.	It is difficult to discuss errors that occur in my daily work.	1	2	3	4	5	X
9.	I am encouraged by my colleagues to report any patient safety concerns I may have.	1	2	3	4	5	X
10.	The culture in the hospital makes it easy to learn from the errors of others.	1	2	3	4	5	X
11.	My suggestions about safety would be acted upon if I expressed them to management.	1	2	3	4	5	X
12.	I am aware of the Housestaff Quality Council.	Yes	■■■■			No	■■■■
13.	This is a good place to work.	1	2	3	4	5	X
14.	Hospital administration supports my daily efforts.	1	2	3	4	5	X
15.	I am aware of the work the Housestaff Quality Council does.	1	2	3	4	5	X
16.	The levels of staffing in my clinical area are sufficient to handle the number of patients.	1	2	3	4	5	X
17.	I am provided with timely information about events in the hospital that might affect my work.	1	2	3	4	5	X
18.	Trainees in my discipline are adequately supervised.	1	2	3	4	5	X
19.	The Housestaff Quality Council communicates well with the housestaff.	1	2	3	4	5	X
20.	I experience good collaboration with attending physicians in my clinical area.	1	2	3	4	5	X
21.	I experience good collaboration with pharmacists in my clinical area.	1	2	3	4	5	X
22.	Communication breakdowns that lead to delays in delivery of care are common.	1	2	3	4	5	X
23.	Communication between housestaff and the hospital regarding patient safety policies is good.	1	2	3	4	5	X
24.	I am provided with timely information by the Housestaff Quality Council about events in the hospital that might affect my work.	1	2	3	4	5	X
25.	My level of knowledge with regards to the dosing of Dilaudid (hydromorphone) has increased over the past year.	1	2	3	4	5	X

I enjoy the quality of teamwork and cooperation/communication with housestaff from: (use the same rating scale as above)

Anesthesiology	1 2 3 4 5 X	Ob/Gyn	1 2 3 4 5 X	Phys Med&Rehab	1 2 3 4 5 X
Dermatology	1 2 3 4 5 X	Ophthalmology	1 2 3 4 5 X	Psychiatry	1 2 3 4 5 X
Emergency Med	1 2 3 4 5 X	Orthopedic Surgery	1 2 3 4 5 X	Rad Oncology	1 2 3 4 5 X
Medicine	1 2 3 4 5 X	Otolaryngology	1 2 3 4 5 X	Radiology	1 2 3 4 5 X
Nephrology	1 2 3 4 5 X	Pathology	1 2 3 4 5 X	Surgery	1 2 3 4 5 X
Neurology	1 2 3 4 5 X	Pediatrics	1 2 3 4 5 X	Urology	1 2 3 4 5 X
Neurosurgery	1 2 3 4 5 X	Plastic Surgery	1 2 3 4 5 X		

Additional Comments to the HQC: _____

_____

Thank you for completing the survey – your time and participation are greatly appreciated.
Disclaimer: This survey is derived from the University of Texas at Austin Copyright 2004 Safety Attitudes in Your Unit and has been modified to address the needs of the NYPH-WCMC.

Fig. 1. New York-Presbyterian-Weill Cornell Medical College Safety Attitude Survey.

Table 1	
Initial safety attitude survey results	
Survey Question	**Score**
It is difficult to speak up if I perceive a problem with patient care.	2.5
It is difficult to discuss errors that occur in my daily work.	2.6
Communication breakdowns that lead to delays in delivery of care are common.	3.0

Scale: 1 = Strongly Disagree; 5 = Strongly Agree.

This survey has also served as a tool to assess the affect of the HQC since its inception. However, it is recognized that the creation of the HQC alone may not be the sole reason for these results; concurrent hospital QPS initiatives may have also influenced the results.

Strategic Plan and Recruitment

With the endorsement of senior leadership to proceed with the formation of the HQC, the residents wrote a letter to each of the clinical department chairmen and program directors, requesting 2 members of the housestaff from each department to join the HQC. Once the housestaff were appointed to the HCQ, the residents put together informational packets that included the presentation to senior leadership, a copy of The Joint Commission National Patient Safety Goals, a communications plan, and a directory of HQC representatives. The first HQC meeting was scheduled, only 5 months after the initial presentation.[4]

First Meeting and Agenda Creation

The first meeting of the HQC took place in April 2008, co-chaired by the residents in anesthesiology. Initially the meetings were focused on a few ideas that would make a difference in quality and safety outcomes. *HOT TOPICS* were discussed, feedback was provided, and various clinical departments were invited to make presentations to the HQC. Through this early format, the HQC representatives developed a list of initiatives that they thought would be most beneficial to improvements in patient care and daily workflow.

The first major QPS initiative that the HQC addressed was immediately following a survey by The Joint Commission. The hospital had received a Requirement for Improvement (RFI) in the area of medication reconciliation and had only 45 days to address its deficiency in compliance. The HQC responded to this need by suggesting that a "hard stop" be placed in the admission order set of the Computerized Provider Order Entry (CPOE) if the medication reconciliation was not performed within the first 12 hours of admission.

Over time, the HQC meetings evolved from passive presentations on QPS initiatives by various departments to HQC-driven discussions of how care can be improved through active participation by the HQC.

Administrative Support

From the outset, the Department of Anesthesiology was instrumental in providing the leadership and administrative support to the HQC and continues to do so today. In addition, the support from the medical school and hospital has been profound, though complex.

The medical director of the CT-ICU serves as the faculty advisor to the HQC and the QPS administrator serves as the QPS liaison. One of the anesthesiology residents who started the HQC was encouraged to focus on the HQC initiatives during his 6-month research elective.

The HQC has received financial support from the senior vice president and chief QPS officer of the Division of Quality and Patient Safety, senior administration, and through grants from the New York-Weill Cornell Center Alumni Council (CAC).

Because of the complexities of the administrative support and relationships, the HQC chair and vice chair meet regularly with senior leadership and the QPS officers to ensure they are well informed about various QPS initiatives at the hospital. One of the challenges is to provide administrative time to the HQC leadership for this purpose. The clinical department chairs have been overwhelmingly supportive of the HQC and with their assistance, they do their best to help the HQC leaders meet these goals while maintaining resident work hour compliance.

Communications

The key to changing culture in any organization is communications among all those involved in the process. The initial conversation between the Department of Anesthesiology and hospital leadership was the first step in this communication process and even more important was the communication between the hospital leadership and the housestaff. If the culture was to change, an effective communication process was needed.

To address the goal of developing a robust, 2-way communications system, the HQC formed a communications subcommittee and identified some of the barriers to effective communications, including the inability for housestaff to identify the importance or relevance of a message.

The HQC engaged Synecticsworld, a company known for its innovative, systematic approach to problem solving, and with their guidance during 4 separate sessions with key members of the HQC, a communications matrix (**Fig. 2**) was established. The

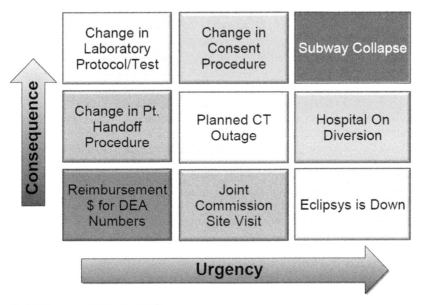

Fig. 2. HQC communications matrix.

matrix is used to prioritize a message as to urgency and consequence and the means of communication is selected based on that priority.[4,6] Some of the methods of communication include e-mail messages, newsletters, posters, alpha-numeric paging, Grand Rounds presentations, and Infonet announcements. In addition, whenever possible, messages are sent directly by the HQC to improve "buy-in."

The HQC also developed a Web site (**Fig. 3**), which is part of the hospital Infonet, dedicated to communications for and about the HQC. They publish a quarterly newsletter, *Clinical Updates*, to summarize the results of recent accomplishments by the HQC.

Resident Quality and Patient Safety Officer

In an effort to recognize the important role of the HQC chair, the chief QPS officer created the role of resident QPS officer in 2009. This position has given the HQC chair an opportunity to learn about the QPS issues at the hospital, to bring these issues back to the HQC in a more enlightened way, and has facilitated alignment with strategic goals between the HQC and the hospital's QPS agenda. Working collaboratively with the other QPS officers at the hospital, the resident QPS officer has helped strengthen the relationship between the HQC and hospital leadership and key clinical and support departments.

Organizational Structure

To ensure a sustainable and functioning organization, the HQC turned its attention to creating formal rules and regulations. A subcommittee was formed to address this topic and the first rules and regulations were ratified by the HQC in May 2009.

The rules and regulations codify the mission and vision of the organization, the composition of the HQC, the responsibilities of the chair and vice chair, the qualifications of the members and their responsibilities, the reappointment process, succession planning, financial authority, and administrative support.

The HQC reports through the hospital's Division of Quality and Patient Safety (**Fig. 4**). The HQC provides periodic reports to the hospital's Medical Board and Board of Trustees Quality and Performance Improvement Committee and is represented on several Medical Board committees, including the QPS Executive Committee, IT Prioritization Committee, Sedation and Analgesia Committee, Perioperative Services Steering Committee, and Surgical Site Infection Committee.

HQC Quality Focus Areas/Alignment with NYP

Each year, quality focus areas are selected by the Division of Quality and Patient Safety with collaboration and approval of hospital leadership. To achieve these goals, it is important for the hospital to foster culture change at the institution and they have emphasized their motto "We Put Patients First" to accomplish this objective.

The hospital has experienced great success with a reduction in central line–associated blood stream infections (CLABSIs), hand hygiene compliance, and other QPS initiatives because of on-going efforts at communications and marketing of its goal: to create a culture of optimal quality and patient safety. At the same time, the HQC has partnered with the hospital in creating synergy with the quality focus areas.

In 2009, the HQC focused its strategic goals to align with those of the hospital. The strategic goals (**Fig. 5**) for the year included medication safety, communications, infection prevention and control, efficiency and patient flow, and surgical and procedural safety. To align with these goals, the HQC established a focus on hydromorphone and morphine sulfate, the communications matrix, compliance with influenza vaccine administration, paperless laboratory orders, and a tracheostomy care checklist.

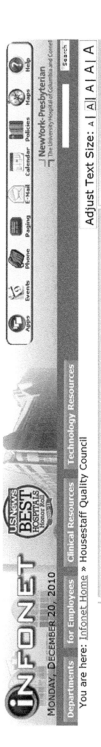
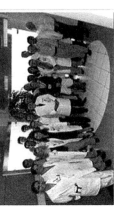

Fig. 3. HQC Infonet Web site.

HQC Structure

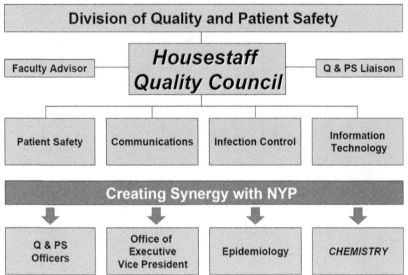

Fig. 4. HQC organizational structure.

Sustainability and Succession Planning

The HQC has continued to develop and grow since it began in 2008. The founding members of the HQC have a vested interest in ensuring that the work of the HQC continues and the ratification of the HQC rules and regulations supports this goal.

In May 2009, in accordance with the rules and regulations, the first election of a vice chair was held and a surgery resident was appointed to the leadership of the HQC for

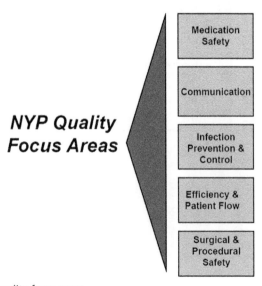

Fig. 5. HQC/NYP quality focus areas.

a 2-year period, first as vice chair, and then as chair for the second year. A second election was held in May 2010 and an internal medicine resident was elected as the 2010–2011 vice chair. With leadership passing outside of the Department of Anesthesiology, the HQC will be sustained by residents from other specialties in medicine.

Replicability

The success of the HQC at NYP has garnered recognition and interest from many other institutions throughout the country and the concept of the HQC has been replicated at other medical centers. In addition, the HQC has been invited to make presentations at the Harvard Quality Colloquium, the ACGME, the American Association of Medical Colleges (AAMC), the David Rogers Health Policy Colloquium, the Duke Physician Leadership in Quality and Patient Safety, the New York State Department of Health, and the American Medical Student Association (AMSA).

RESULTS

How has the HQC improved quality and patient safety? By forging a bi-directional communication pathway with senior leadership and key clinical and administrative departments, thereby developing a systematic approach to identifying QPS issues where housestaff participation will affect outcomes. This approach includes (1) identifying QPS issues, (2) collecting data, (3) analyzing data, (4) implementing process/system changes, and (5) monitoring the effectiveness of the changes.

Over the past 3 years, the HQC has made several important contributions to QPS improvements, some of which are highlighted as follows:

1. Medication Reconciliation: As previously mentioned, this Joint Commission National Patient Safety Goal requirement was championed by a group of HQC members after receiving an RFI during a Joint Commission accreditation site visit. With 45 days to develop a corrective action plan, the HQC recommended placing hard stops in the electronic medical record admission order set and worked collaboratively with Nursing and Information Technology to accomplish this. Once this force function was placed in the CPOE system, compliance increased to 90% or greater, which was sustained when re-measured at 6 months (**Fig. 6**).[7] This initiative was successful because it engaged all housestaff in the policy and decision-making process and raised awareness of the need for immediate compliance. In

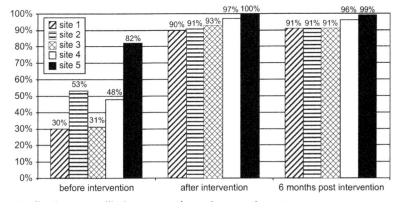

Fig. 6. Medication reconciliation pre- and post-intervention rates.

addition, since this was a housestaff-driven solution, the housestaff became the communicators and enforcers of complying with medication reconciliation.

2. Changing Physician Behavior, through close collaboration with the hospital's QPS officers, has afforded the HQC an opportunity to recommend substantive changes in the processes and systems that enhance patient safety. As an example of this, the HQC focused on hydromorphone-related respiratory depression. Hydromorphone is 7 times more potent than morphine and reduced hydromorphone doses can achieve the same analgesic effect as morphine. The HQC sought to limit dose ranges for hydromorphone. One of the National Quality Forum (NQF) Never Events, defined as an inexcusable outcome in a health care setting, is death or disability associated with a medication error.[8] This initiative was accomplished by placing a constraint or force function in the hospital's CPOE system, whereby the prescribing dose range was limited. A 50% reduction in higher doses was realized in just 1 month of the CPOE change (**Fig. 7**). Pain scores, medical event reporting, and naloxone usage is being analyzed to show evidence of effectiveness

3. Use of the Electronic Medical Record to Improve Accuracy of Lab Ordering was initiated with a goal of having all lab tests ordered through the CPOE system to decrease lab ordering errors; ensure correct patient identification, blood tube selection, and labeling; reduce duplicate orders; effectively track missing lab specimens; and most importantly, reduce the results turnaround time back to housestaff. This collaborative project was conducted with Nursing and the Department of Pathology. After orienting physicians to the benefits of electronic ordering of lab tests, and providing the necessary technical support, a 75% decrease from baseline was realized in all ICUs over a 7-month period (**Fig. 8**).

4. A Patient Safety Awareness Campaign was launched in July 2009 to encourage transparency in reporting medical errors and to promote vigilance in identifying possible flaws in hospital processes and systems. Areas highlighted included deep vein thrombosis prophylaxis, potency of hydromorphone (Dilaudid) versus morphine sulfate, retained central line guidewires, electronic order entry, antibiotic

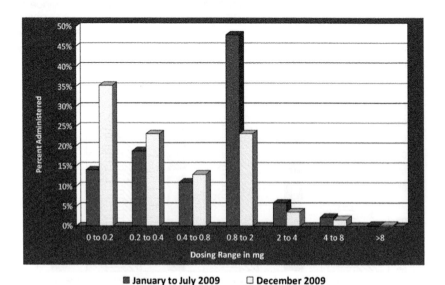

■ January to July 2009   ☐ December 2009

Fig. 7. Changes in hydromorphone prescribing.

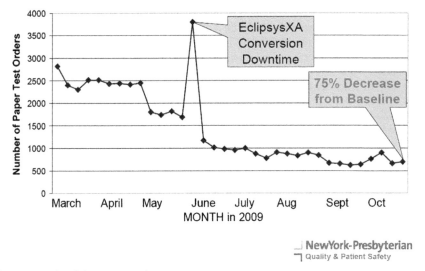

Fig. 8. Paperless laboratory project.

administration in sepsis, insulin management, excessive lab ordering, checking labs before central line placement, and not seeking help.[4,9]

Additional initiatives have been undertaken by the HQC including development of a standardized tracheostomy care checklist, improvement in vaccination rates in eligible patients, proper collection and submission of tissue samples, creation of an opiate conversion card, and an emergency code lab order set.

SUMMARY

In 2005, the American Society of Anesthesiology (ASA) published a report "Task Force on Future Paradigms of Anesthesia Practice," which asserted that the field of anesthesiology was uniquely positioned to be a clinical and administrative leader in tertiary care hospitals.[10] At the 2006 American Society of Anesthesiologists (ASA) Annual Meeting, Mark A. Warner, MD, built on this concept when delivering the 44th Annual Rovenstine keynote lecture. Dr Warner suggested that for anesthesiologists to embrace their changing role in health care systems, residency programs must improve the preparation of trainees in health care administration so they are prepared to explore opportunities to advance various aspects of health care.[11]

Simultaneously, many other national organizations were focusing on how to engage housestaff in quality and patient safety to improve the current quality of care delivered. Specifically, the ACGME, the Alliance for Independent Academic Medical Centers (AIAMC), the AAMC, and the Lucian Leape Institute, released white papers, launched initiatives, and/or held national conferences in the past 5 years focused on this concept.[12–15]

Conceived and initiated by the Department of Anesthesiology at NYP Hospital, Weill Cornell Medical Center, the HQC illustrates one model that both engages housestaff in QPS while simultaneously creating future leaders in this area. Although the HQC and department have garnered a good deal of recognition over the 3-year period since its inception, they still face barriers to success. These include (1) defining the optimal means of communication that will involve housestaff in new policies and procedures,

(2) creating a balance between transparency in reporting measured safety and quality indicators and hospital confidentiality, (3) measuring a culture change despite perception of its success, and (4) creating protected time for housestaff to perform administrative duties while recognizing the primary goal of residency education and clinical experience.

The field of anesthesiology has a long tradition of quality improvement and patient safety. In 1985, it became the first medical specialty to create a separate foundation, the Anesthesia Patient Safety Foundation (APSF), specifically focused on improving patient safety and reducing morbidity caused by anesthesia administration. In 2009, the ASA launched the Anesthesia Quality Institute (AQI), a national registry developed to collect data for the assessment and improvement of anesthesia care. The ultimate goal of the AQI is (1) to serve as a resource to anesthesiologists to obtain patient safety and quality management data and (2) to help anesthesiologists meet regulatory requirements designed to improve patient care.[16]

Given the longstanding commitment to improving and fostering innovation in patient safety, anesthesiologists are well poised to involve housestaff in these initiatives, thereby providing an opportunity to initiate a system-wide culture change and nurture future leaders in this area.

REFERENCES

1. Accreditation Council for Graduate Medical Education. ACGME Fact Sheet. Available at: http://www.acgme.org/acWebsite/newsRoom/newsRm_factSheet.asp. Accessed July 29, 2010.
2. 2008–2018 National employment matrix, bureau of labor statistics.
3. Kerr G, Fleischut P, Evans A, et al. Anesthesiology department creates innovative council to promote patient safety at their hospital. ASA Newsl 2009;73(9):32–3.
4. Fleischut P, Evans A, Nugent W, et al. Ten Years after the IOM Report: engaging residents in quality and patient safety by creating a housestaff quality council. American Journal of Medical Quality in press.
5. Fleischut P, Evans A, Kerr G, et al. Engaging housestaff in quality improvement and patient safety at an academic medical institution. New York: System Quality Review; 2008. p. 65–7.
6. Nugent W, Fleischut P, Kerr G, et al. Housestaff communication processes improvements: matching the message to the medium. New York: System quality review; 2009. p. 78–80.
7. Evans A, Lazar E, Tiase V, et al. The role of housestaff in implementing medication reconciliation on admission at an academic medical center. Published online before print. Am J Med Qual 2010. [Epub ahead of print].
8. Patient Care Primer. Never events. Agency for healthcare research and quality. Available at: http://www.psnet.ahrq.gov/primer.aspx?primerID=3. Accessed July 29, 1010.
9. Fleischut P, Nugent W, Kerr G, et al. Novel approach to preventing housestaff medical errors. System Quality Review 2009;10:76–7.
10. Miller RD. Report from the task force on future paradigms of anesthesia practice. ASA Newsl 2005;69:2–6.
11. Warner MA. Who better than anesthesiologists? The 44th Rovenstine Lecture. Anesthesiology 2006;104:1094–101.
12. Philibert I. Involving residents in quality improvement: contrasting top-down and bottom-up approaches. Accreditation Council for Graduate Medical Education and the Institute for Healthcare Improvement 90-day project. August 2008.

Available at: http://www.acgme.org/acWebsite/ci/90DayProjectReportDFA_PA_09_15_08.pdf. Accessed July 29, 2010.

13. National Initiative (NI). Improving patient care through GME. Alliance for Independent Academic Medical Centers. Available at: http://www.aiamc.org. Accessed July 29, 2010.

14. Association of American Medical Colleges. Integrating quality: linking clinical and educational excellence. Chicago, June 3–4, 2010. Available at: http://www.aamc.org/meetings/opiquality/2010/start.htm. Accessed July 29, 2010.

15. Unmet Needs. Teaching physicians to provide safe patient care. Report of the Lucian Leape Institute Roundtable on Reforming Medical Education. Boston; March 2010. Available at: http://www.npsf.org/download/LLI-Unmet-Needs-Report.pdf. Accessed July 29, 2010.

16. The Anesthesia Quality Institute (AQI) and The National Anesthesia Clinical Outcomes Registry (NACOR). Available at: http://www.aqihq.org/Introduction.aspx. Accessed July 29, 2010.

Index

Note: Page numbers of article titles are in **boldface** type.

A

Acute pain, outcomes assessment of evidence-based guidelines and registries, 124–125

Adverse event tracking, improved, with anesthesia information management systems, 61

Aging. *See* Geriatrics.

American College of Surgeons National Surgical Quality Improvement Program, 74–75

Anesthesia care, quality of, 1–167

    cultural change at a hospital system level, **153–167**

    effect of teamwork and communication in the OR on outcomes, **1–11**

        discussion, 4–10

        study methods, 2

        study results, 2–4

    in pain management, **123–133**

    medication safety in the perioperative period, **135–144**

    multidisciplinary education to improve, **99–110**

    outcomes research using quality improvement databases, **71–81**

    preventing postoperative complications in the elderly, **83–97**

    promoting palliative care in the ICU, **111–122**

    reduction of regulated medical waste, **145–152**

    simulation and quality improvement, **13–28**

        clinical outcomes, 19–20

        educational outcomes, 15–18

        features of high-quality simulators, 14–15

        for identifying latent errors, 20–21

        for maintenance of certification in anesthesiology, 22

        history of simulators, 14–15

        skills transfer, 18–19

        translational research, 14

    using information technology to improve, **29–55**

    using real-time clinical decision support to improve, **57–69**

Anesthesia information management systems (AIMS), for real-time clinical decision support, **57–69**

    decision support to improve quality based on, 62–65

        cost-effectiveness, 65

        detection of outliers, 65

        improving quality of information transfer, 65

        operational, 63–64

        reminders for adherence to clinical guidelines, 62–63

    event reporting and tracking to improve quality, 60–62

        improvements in adverse event tracking, 61

        improvements in data capture and record quality, 60–61

Anesthesiology Clin 29 (2011) 169–178

doi:10.1016/S1932-2275(11)00009-7

1932-2275/11/$ – see front matter © 2011 Elsevier Inc. All rights reserved.

Erratum

In the article, "Sugammadex: Cyclodextrins, Development of Selective Binding Agents, Pharmacology, Clinical Development, and Future Directions," by Sadighi Akha et al, in the 28:4 issue of *Anesthesiology Clinics*, there was an error in reference #34; the location of the abstract presented was incorrect. The correct reference is: Soto R, Jahr JS, Pavlin J, Sabo D, Morte JB. Safety and efficacy of sugammadex reversal of rocuronium-induced block versus spontaneous recovery from succinylcholine. Presented at the New York State Society of Anesthesiologists Post Graduate Assembly in December 2010, New York, NY.

Anesthesiology Clin 29 (2011) I
doi:10.1016/j.anclin.2010.12.003
1932-2275/11/$ – see front matter © 2011 Elsevier Inc. All rights reserved.
anesthesiology.theclinics.com

Moving?

Make sure your subscription moves with you!

To notify us of your new address, find your **Clinics Account Number** (located on your mailing label above your name), and contact customer service at:

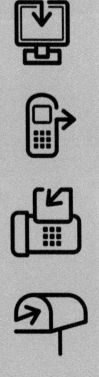

Email: journalscustomerservice-usa@elsevier.com

800-654-2452 (subscribers in the U.S. & Canada)
314-447-8871 (subscribers outside of the U.S. & Canada)

Fax number: 314-447-8029

Elsevier Health Sciences Division
Subscription Customer Service
3251 Riverport Lane
Maryland Heights, MO 63043

*To ensure uninterrupted delivery of your subscription, please notify us at least 4 weeks in advance of move.

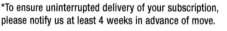

Printed and bound by CPI Group (UK) Ltd, Croydon, CR0 4YY

03/10/2024

01040460-0019